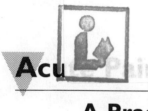

Acu ... t

A Pra

D0714665

This book is due for return on or before the last date shown below.

27 NOV 1997	31.7.09	

Important notice

Every effort has been made to check the drug dosages given in this book. However, as it is possible that dosage schedules have been revised, the reader is strongly urged to consult the drug companies' literature before administering any of the drugs listed.

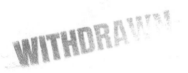

Acute Pain Management

A Practical Guide

♦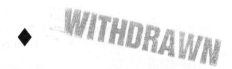

PAMELA E MACINTYRE, BMEDSC, MBBS, FANZCA,
Director Acute Pain Service,
Department of Anaesthesia and Intensive Care,
Royal Adelaide Hospital and University of Adelaide,
Adelaide, Australia
and
L BRIAN READY, MD, FRCP(C),
Professor, Department of Anesthesiology,
Director, UWMC Pain Service,
University of Washington, Seattle, USA

With contributions from:
Judith R Atkins, RN,
RN Coordinator, Acute Pain Service,
Royal Adelaide Hospital,
Adelaide, Australia
and
Lorie Wild, RN, MN,
Clinical Nurse Specialist in Pain,
University of Washington Medical Center,
Seattle, USA

W.B. Saunders Company Ltd
London • Philadelphia • Toronto
Sydney • Tokyo

W.B. Saunders Company Ltd 24–28 Oval Road
London NW1 7DX

The Curtis Center
Independence Square West
Philadelphia, PA 19106–3399, USA

Harcourt Brace & Company
55 Horner Avenue
Toronto, Ontario M8Z 4X6, Canada

Harcourt Brace & Company, Australia
30–52 Smidmore Street
Marrickville, NSW 2204, Australia

Harcourt Brace & Company, Japan
Ichibancho Central Building
22–1 Ichibancho
Chiyoda-ku, Tokyo 102, Japan

A catalogue record for this book is available from the British Library

ISBN 0–7020–1990–9

Typeset by J&L Composition Ltd, Filey, North Yorkshire
Printed and bound in Great Britain by WBC Book Manufacturers Ltd,
Bridgend, Mid Glamorgan

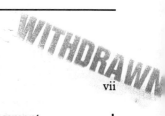

CONTENTS

O ver the last decade exciting new techniques of acute pain management have been introduced, studied and incorporated into clinical practice. Patient-controlled analgesia and epidural analgesia, for example, have been revolutionary. In many hospitals, acute pain teams have emerged to facilitate the use of these special techniques. Such teams typically consist of physicians with a special interest and expertise in pain management who collaborate with nurses who have acquired new skills and knowledge at the bedside in order to bring to their patients the benefits of effective and safe analgesia. Junior medical staff will benefit from a sound understanding of these newer analgesic techniques although in many settings they will not be directly responsible for using them.

Not all patients have or need access to these newer methods of pain relief. However, for these patients, pain management using older and more conventional methods, such as intermittent intramuscular injections of opioid, has improved very little. The responsibility for the management of these forms of analgesia is often delegated to junior medical and nursing staff who have had insufficient experience or appropriate education to enable them to use these methods of pain relief with optimal effect.

Essential to better treatment of pain, whether simple or sophisticated forms of analgesia are used, is a good understanding of the drugs and techniques available, a team approach to the problem and a good working relationship between all members of the health care team and the patient. Together, these groups can play a major role in improving the effectiveness and safety of all methods of pain relief.

The aim of the book is to provide nurses, medical students and doctors in training (interns, house officers, residents and registrars) with simple and practical information and guidelines for the safe and more effective management of conventional methods of analgesia and to give them an understanding of the newer techniques available for the treatment of acute pain in adults. It is also hoped that the book may be of use to other general and specialist medical practitioners with an interest in the treatment of acute pain, especially those about to introduce changes to the way acute pain is managed in their institution.

As a practical book only, information about the anatomy, neurochemistry and pathophysiology of acute pain has been omitted. A section on pain relief in specific situations has not been included as good analgesia should be possible for most if not all patients if the basic principles of acute pain management are understood.

It is not possible for a book of this size to contain detailed information on every drug and every technique used for the management of acute pain and only those in common use in the USA, Australia and the UK have been included. Suggested drugs, doses and treatment regimens are guidelines only and may vary according to different hospitals and different patient populations.

Pamela E Macintrye
L. Brian Ready

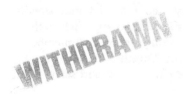

CHAPTER I

ACUTE PAIN: SIGNIFICANCE AND ASSESSMENT

◆

Harmful effects of undertreated acute pain;

Results of better management of acute pain;

Recommendations for improved management of acute pain;

Acute pain services;

Definition of pain;

Measurement of pain

Since the 1960s a number of studies of adult hospital patients have highlighted inadequacies in the treatment of acute pain. In the postoperative period up to 75% of patients have reported moderate to severe pain. Patients with other causes of acute pain, such as burns, multiple trauma, renal colic and myocardial infarction, have fared no better. One of the main reasons often cited for poor analgesia is the lack of knowledge that nursing and medical staff have about the drugs and their methods of administration. Inadequate education, combined with some of the many myths associated with pain management, has resulted in suboptimal analgesia for many patients. These myths have included:

- 'pain is not harmful to the patient'
- 'pain relief obscures the signs of surgical complications'
- 'the patient will become addicted to opioids'
- 'the risk of respiratory depression with opioids is high'
- 'patient weight is the best predictor of opioid requirement'
- 'the maximum dose of an opioid is the contents of one ampule'
- 'opioids must not be given more often than 4-hourly'
- 'PRN means "give as infrequently as possible" or "not on my shift!"'

More recently there have been significant improvements in the management of acute pain. These improvements have largely been due to the introduction of new techniques for the delivery of analgesic drugs, such as patient-controlled analgesia and epidural analgesia and a growing interest among anesthesiologists. Pain management for patients dependent on more conventional techniques, such as intermittent intramuscular opioid analgesia, has improved little if at all.

HARMFUL EFFECTS OF UNDERTREATED ACUTE PAIN

It was often thought that even if pain was not good for the patient at least it did no harm. It is now recognized that undertreatment of severe acute pain can have a number of harmful physiological and psychological effects (**Box 1.1**).

Possible harmful effects of undertreated severe acute pain	
Respiratory	Decreased lung volumes, atelectasis, decreased cough, sputum retention, infection, hypoxemia
Cardiovascular	Tachycardia, hypertension, increased peripheral vascular resistance, increased myocardial oxygen consumption, myocardial ischemia, altered regional blood flow, deep vein thrombosis
Gastrointestinal	Decreased gastric and bowel motility
Genitourinary	Urinary retention
Neuroendocrine	Increases in the levels of catecholamines, cortisol, glucagon, growth hormone, vasopressin, aldosterone and insulin
Psychological	Anxiety, fear, sleeplessness
Musculoskeletal	Muscle spasm, immobility (increasing risk of deep vein thrombosis)

Box 1.1

EFFECTS ON THE RESPIRATORY SYSTEM

Pain from operation or injury to the chest or abdomen can exaggerate postoperative pulmonary dysfunction, resulting in splinting of the muscles of the diaphragm and chest wall and a reduced ability to cough. This leads to a reduction in lung volumes (tidal volume, vital capacity, forced expiratory volume and functional residual capacity), atelectasis and sputum retention, which can result in hypoxemia and an increased risk of chest infections.

EFFECTS ON THE CARDIOVASCULAR SYSTEM

Severe pain increases sympathetic nervous system activity, resulting in rises in heart rate, blood pressure and peripheral vascular resistance. These in turn increase the workload of the heart and the oxygen consumption of the myocardium. Myocardial oxygen supply may already be decreased owing to cardiac or respiratory disease or as a result of hypoxemia from the postoperative pulmonary changes outlined above. If oxygen consumption is greater than oxygen supply, myocardial ischemia (which, in the postoperative period, may be silent) will result.

Increased sympathetic stimulation may also alter regional blood flow, directing blood away from viscera towards brain and heart. Decreased blood flow may impair wound healing and increase muscle spasm.

Severe pain may reduce patient mobility and promote venous stasis. Increases in fibrinogen and platelet activation (see below) will increase blood coagulability. Both of these factors will increase the risk of deep vein thrombosis and pulmonary embolism.

EFFECTS ON THE GASTROINTESTINAL AND GENITOURINARY SYSTEMS

Pain can lead to significant delays in gastric emptying, a reduction in gut motility and urinary retention.

EFFECTS ON THE NEUROENDOCRINE AND METABOLIC SYSTEMS

Pain is believed to play a major part in the activation of the neuroendocrine 'stress response' seen after surgery or trauma and resulting in the release of a number of hormones (see **Box 1.1**). These changes can lead to hyperglycemia, increases in fibrinogen and platelet activation (increased coagulability), increased protein breakdown and a negative nitrogen balance, and impairment of both wound healing and immune function (with a consequent decreased resistance to infection). Insulin levels, low during surgery, are increased in the postoperative period but are not adequate to control the hyperglycemia that develops. Sodium and water retention may also occur.

PSYCHOLOGICAL EFFECTS

Untreated pain can lead to or increase patient anxiety, fear and sleeplessness. Aggressive or belligerent behaviour may be a sign of anxiety and distress.

OTHER EFFECTS

Muscle spasm may further reduce respiratory function and immobility will increase the possibility of venous stasis and deep vein thrombosis.

Adding to these effects may be other factors related to the injury or operation causing the pain. For example, decreases in lung volume will also be seen in the presence of abdominal distension resulting from ileus or ascites.

RESULTS OF BETTER MANAGEMENT OF ACUTE PAIN

Analgesia can at least partially reverse some of the harmful effects of untreated, severe acute pain. Thus, effective treatment of acute pain is important not only for the humanitarian reasons of patient comfort and satisfaction, but because it can significantly improve outcome, especially in the high-risk patient.

For example, a study by Yeager et al (1987) showed that in high risk surgical patients, the better pain relief provided by epidural analgesia compared with conventional methods of analgesia resulted in a decreased incidence of postoperative cardiac and respiratory complications, less infection and a lower overall cost per patient. Rawal et al (1984), comparing epidural and conventional analgesia in patients after gastroplasty, noted earlier mobilization, fewer pulmonary complications, earlier return of bowel function and a decrease in the average length of stay in hospital in the epidural group. When patient-controlled analgesia (PCA) was compared with intramuscular morphine analgesia after hysterectomy, Wasylak et al (1990) demonstrated that patients with PCA not only were more comfortable but also were able to mobilize and eat before patients in the other group and had a shorter stay in hospital.

RECOMMENDATIONS FOR IMPROVED MANAGEMENT OF ACUTE PAIN

There has been a gradual increase in the recognition of the need for better acute pain management. In the last few years major bodies worldwide have lent their support to this recognition and have published recommendations and guidelines aimed at improving the treatment of acute pain. These have included:

1. **The Royal College of Surgeons of England and the College of Anaesthetists**: their *Report of the Working Party on Pain after Surgery* makes a number of recommendations for the improvement of postoperative pain relief. These include the need for better education of all staff; systematic assessment and recording of pain; acute pain teams to be established in all major hospitals; the introduction of new methods of pain relief and the improved use of existing methods; continuous audit of activity; and the provision of appropriate staff and facilities for these services (Royal College of Surgeons and College of Anaesthetists, 1990).

2. **Faculty of Anaesthetists and Royal Australasian College of Surgeons**: their *Statement on Acute Pain Management* contains similar recommendations for the improvement of the management of acute pain (Faculty of Anaesthetists and Royal Australasian College of Surgeons, 1991).

3. **International Association for the Study of Pain (IASP)**:

the IASP Task Force on Acute Pain released *Management of Acute Pain: A Practical Guide*, which deals with the practical aspects of improving the treatment of acute pain, (Ready and Edwards, 1992).

4. **US Department of Health and Human Services, Agency for Health Care Policy and Research (AHCPR)**: the AHCPR *Clinical Practice Guideline* for acute pain management was developed by a multidisciplinary independent panel whose recommendations were based primarily on the published literature. As well as explanations of the need for better control of pain and guidelines for the use of the various analgesic options available, the publication recommends a team approach to pain control (including the patient); frequent assessment of the patient's pain; and a 'formal approach to the management of acute pain, with clear lines of responsibility' (Carr et al, 1992).

5. **American Society of Anesthesiologists (ASA)**: the report of the ASA Task Force on Acute Pain Management contains recommendations similar to those of the Royal College of Surgeons of England, designed to improve postoperative pain management. It emphasizes the benefits of a formal interdisciplinary individualized approach to pain control using both drug and non-drug treatments, and the responsibilities that institutions have to provide the best pain relief for their patients (Ready et al, 1995).

These reports stress that a patient has the right to expect adequate treatment of pain and that all members of the health care team have an ethical obligation to provide it. The ethical importance is further increased when additional benefits such as improved outcome are considered.

Common to these reports is the recommendation that all major acute care centers should establish acute pain teams or acute pain services. In centers where there are no pain management teams, it is recommended that responsibility for effective and safe analgesia be taken by a named member of staff.

ACUTE PAIN SERVICES

The first acute pain service was started in 1986 at the University of Washington in Seattle. Since that time many hospitals worldwide have followed suit. The main medical member of the team is often an anesthesiologist because the knowledge required and many of the techniques used are simply extensions of those employed in the operating room. An acute pain service has a unique opportunity not only to introduce and manage the newer techniques now available for acute pain management, but also to participate in the education of all medical and nursing staff and patients and provide information and advice about the more effective use of the older and more conventional methods of analgesia.

In order to do this effectively, an organized team approach is important. Suggestions for this organization are summarized in the American Society of Anesthesiologists guidelines (**Box 1.2**).

DEFINITION OF PAIN

The International Association for the Study of Pain defines pain as

> *'An unpleasant sensory and emotional experience associated with actual or potential tissue damage or described in terms of such damage.'*

Pain is a very individual experience, and many factors including previous pain experiences, cultural background, disease or surgical prognosis, coping strategies, fear, anxiety and depression, will interact to produce what the patient then describes as pain. Not surprisingly, there is often a poor correlation between the patient's assessment of the pain and the nursing or medical staff's estimate of the pain that the patient is experiencing.

Organizational aspects of an anesthesiology-based postoperative pain program

1. *Education (initial, updates):*
   anesthesiologists
   surgeons
   nurses
   pharmacists
   patients and families
   hospital administrators
   health insurance carriers
2. *Areas of regular administrative activity:*
   maintenance of clear lines of communication
   manpower – 24-hour availability of pain service personnel
   evaluation (including safety) of equipment (e.g. pumps)
   secretarial support
   economic issues
   continuous quality improvement (CQI)
   resident physician teaching (if applicable)
   pain management-related research (if applicable)
3. *Collaboration with nursing services:*
   job description of pain service nurse (if applicable)
   nursing policies and procedures
   nurses in-service and continuing education
   definition of roles in patient care
   institutional administrative activities
   continuous quality improvement (CQI)
   research activities (if applicable)
4. *Elements of documentation:*
   preprinted orders
   procedures
   protocols
   bedside pain management flow sheets
   daily consultation notes
   educational packages

Box 1.2
Reproduced from Ready et al (1995) with permission

MEASUREMENT OF PAIN

There are a number of simple clinical techniques available for the assessment and measurement of pain and its response to treatment. The best methods involve self-reporting by the patient rather than observer assessment. Observation of behavior and vital signs is a very unreliable measure of pain and should not be used to assess pain unless the patient is unable to communicate. Discrepancies between a patient's behavior and the self-report of pain may result from differences in coping skills.

In adults, three common methods of self-reported pain measurement are the visual analog scale, the verbal numerical rating scale and the categorical rating scale. Each of these methods of measurement is reasonably reliable as long as the endpoints and adjectives employed are carefully selected and standardized.

While often used to compare levels of pain between patients, these methods are probably of most use as a measure of changes in the level of pain within each patient and the effectiveness of the treatment of that pain.

VISUAL ANALOG SCALE

The visual analog scale (VAS) uses a 10-cm line with endpoint descriptors such as 'no pain' marked at the left end of the line and 'worst pain imaginable' marked at the right end (Figure 1.1). There are no other cues marked on the line. Patients are asked to mark a point on the line that best represents their pain. The distance from 'no pain' to the patient's mark is then measured and this equals the VAS score.

To simplify this measurement, VAS slide rules have been developed. On the front of the slide rule is a 10-cm line with the endpoints such as 'no pain' and 'worst pain imaginable'. The reverse side of the slide rule shows the same line marked at

No pain   Worst pain imaginable

Figure 1.1
Visual analog pain scale

millimeter intervals. The patient moves the slide along the line on the front of the slide rule to the point that best represents their pain. The corresponding VAS measurement is then read off the back of the slide rule.

The disadvantages of the VAS system are that it can be more time-consuming than other simple scoring methods, specific equipment is needed (albeit very simple equipment) and some patients may have difficulty understanding or performing this score, especially in the immediate postoperative period. One advantage of this method is that the wording can be written in many different languages.

The VAS can also be adapted to measure other subjective variables such as patient satisfaction, pain relief and nausea.

VERBAL NUMERICAL RATING SCALE

The verbal numerical rating scale (VNRS) is very similar to the VAS. Patients are asked to imagine that '0 equals no pain' and '10 equals the worst pain imaginable' and then to give a number on this scale that would best represent their pain. The advantage of this type of system is that it does not require any equipment. However, problems may occur if there is a language barrier or the patient has some other difficulty in understanding the scoring system.

With both the VAS and VNRS methods there can be considerable interpatient variation in what is considered to be a 'comfortable' score. For example, for one patient 'comfort' may be a score of 1 or 2, whereas another patient may claim to be very comfortable but give a score of 4 or 5. This highlights the possible problems that can arise if titration of analgesic medication is carried out according to particular pain scores only. Where there is uncertainty, it can be more helpful simply to ask patients whether they are comfortable and satisfied with their current pain therapy.

There has been shown to be a good correlation between the VAS and VNRS methods of measuring pain.

CATEGORICAL RATING SCALE

Other systems of pain measurement use different words to rate pain, such as *none, mild, moderate, severe, very severe* and *worst pain imaginable.*

It is usually not possible, practical or safe to aim for complete pain relief at all times with most of the drugs and drug administration techniques currently available. The aim of treatment should be patient comfort, both at rest and with movement or coughing.

WHEN SHOULD PAIN BE MEASURED?

Patients are usually asked to rate their pain when they are resting. However, a better indicator of the effectiveness of analgesia is an assessment of the pain caused by coughing, deep breathing or movement (e.g. turning in bed).

Pain should be reassessed regularly during the postoperative period. The frequency of assessment should be increased if the pain is poorly controlled or if the pain stimulus or treatment interventions are changing.

REFERENCES AND FURTHER READING

Carr D.B., Jacox A.K., Chapman R.C. et al. (1992) *Acute Pain Management: Operative or Medical Procedures and Trauma, Clinical Practice Guideline.* AHCPR Pub. No. 92-0032. Rockville, MD: Agency for Health Care Policy and Research, Public Health Service, US Department of Health and Human Services.

Faculty of Anaesthetists and Royal Australasian College of Surgeons. (1991) *Statement on Acute Pain Management.* Melbourne.

Macintyre P.E., Runciman W.B.R. and Webb R.K. (1990) An acute pain service in an Australian teaching hospital – the first year. *Medical Journal of Australia* **153**, 417–420.

Murphy D.F., McDonald A., Power C., Unwin A. and MacSullivan R. (1988) Measurement of pain: a comparison of the visual analogue with a nonvisual analogue scale. *Clinical Journal of Pain* **3**, 197–199.

Phillips G.D. and Cousins M.J.C. (1986) Neurological mechanisms of pain and the relationship of pain, anxiety and sleep. In *Acute Pain Management* (eds Phillips G.D. and Cousins M.J.C.). Churchill Livingstone, New York.

Rawal N., Sjöstrand U., Christoffersson E., Dahlström B., Arvill A. and Rydman H. (1984) Comparison of intramuscular and epidural morphine for postoperative analgesia in the grossly obese: influence on postoperative ambulation and pulmonary function. *Anesthesia and Analgesia* **63**, 583–592.

Ready L.B.and Edwards W.T. (eds) (1992) *Management of Acute Pain: A Practical Guide.* IASP Publications, Seattle.

Ready L.B., Oden R., Chadwick H.S., Benedetti C., Rooke G.A., Caplan R. and Wilde L.M. (1988) Development of an anesthesiology-based postoperative pain management service. *Anesthesiology* **68**, 100–106.

Ready L.B., Ashburn M., Caplan R.A., Carr D.B., Connis, R.T., Dixon C.L., Hubbard L. and Rice L.J. (1995) Practice Guidelines for Acute Pain Management in the Perioperative Setting – a report of the American Society of Anesthesiologists Task Force on Pain Management, Acute Pain Section. *Anesthesiology* **82**: 1071–1081.

Royal College of Surgeons and College of Anaesthetists. (1990) Commission on the Provision of Surgical Services. *Report of the Working Party on Pain After Surgery.* London.

Sinatra R.S. (1992) Pathophysiology of acute pain. In *Acute Pain – Mechanisms and Management* (eds Sinatra R.S., Hord A.H., Ginsberg B. and Preble L.M.). Mosby Year Book, St Louis.

Wasylak T.J., Abbott F.V., English M.J.M. and Jeans M.E. (1990) Reduction of postoperative morbidity following patient-controlled morphine. *Canadian Journal of Anaesthesia* **37**, 726–731.

Wheatley R.J., Madej T.H., Jackson I.J.B. and Hunter D. (1991) The first year's experience of an acute pain service. *British Journal of Anaesthesia* **67**, 353–359.

Weissman C. (1990) The metabolic response to stress: an overview and update. *Anesthesiology* **73**, 308–327.

Yeager M.P., Glass D.D., Neff R.K. and Brinck-Johnsen T. (1987) Epidural anesthesia and analgesia in high-risk surgical patients. *Anesthesiology* **66**, 729–736.

CHAPTER 2

PHARMACOLOGY OF OPIOIDS

Opioid receptors and endogenous opioids;
Side effects of opioids;
Predictors of opioid dose;
Titration of opioid dose;
Equianalgesic doses of opioid drugs;
Opioid agonists;
Partial agonists and agonist-antagonists;
Opioid antagonists;
Opioid tolerance, dependence and
addiction

Opium contains some 25 different alkaloids. Only two of these have any analgesic action – morphine (10% by weight of opium) and codeine (0.5% by weight). These naturally occurring substances are called *opiates*. All drugs that have morphine-like actions, naturally occurring or synthetic, are called *opioids*. The term *narcotic*, nowadays, is probably best confined to a more legal sense referring to drugs capable of producing dependence.

In one of its many forms or preparations, opium has been used for the treatment of pain for over two thousand years. The psychological effects of opium were known for hundreds of years before that, and reference is made to its analgesic effects in Egyptian mythology; however, the first accepted reference to its use for the treatment of pain is found in the writings of Theophrastus in the third century BC. Traditionally, opium is obtained from the unripe seed capsule of the poppy *Papaver somniferum*, but this method of collection is very labor-intensive. An alternative and more modern method of production harvests the dried poppy, separates the crop into seeds and straw and extracts morphine, codeine and thebaine from the poppy straw.

In 1806 Sertürner isolated an alkaloid of opium, later called morphine (after Morpheus – the Greek god of dreams and son of Hypnos, god of sleep). The introduction of the hypodermic injection using a glass syringe and hollow needle in 1853 undoubtedly facilitated the use of morphine, but also its abuse. The recognition that morphine was potentially addictive stimulated a search, so far unsuccessful, for other potent but nonaddicting opioids. Unfortunately, the fear of addiction has been a major factor in the undertreatment of acute pain.

OPIOID RECEPTORS AND ENDOGENOUS OPIOIDS

Until the mid-1970s little was known about the mechanism of action of opioid drugs. Since then, not only have receptor sites for these drugs been identified but it was discovered that the body is also capable of producing its own endogenous opioids. In 1973 opioid receptors were identified in the brain and spinal cord, and in 1975 endogenous opioids were isolated.

ENDOGENOUS OPIOIDS
The endogenous opioids identified so far are *endorphins*, *enkephalins* and *dynorphins*. They are found in the brain, spinal cord, gastrointestinal tract and plasma, and are released in response to stimuli such as pain or stress.

OPIOID RECEPTORS
Opioids produce their effect by binding to opioid receptors located in the brain and spinal cord. To date, a number of different opioid receptor types have been identified – mu (μ), delta (δ), kappa (κ) and sigma (σ). Two types of μ receptors, μ_1 and μ_2, have been proposed, with subtype μ_1 mediating analgesia and μ_2 responsible for respiratory depression. All currently avail-

able μ receptor agonist opioids activate both subtypes. The effects of activation of the different receptors are summarized in **Box 2.1.**

According to their action on the opioid receptors, opioid drugs are classed as:

- *agonists*: drugs that bind to and stimulate opioid receptors and are capable of producing a maximal response from the receptor
- *antagonists*: drugs that bind to but do not stimulate opioid receptors and may reverse the effect of opioid agonists
- *partial agonists*: drugs that stimulate opioid receptors but have a ceiling effect, i.e. produce a submaximal response compared with an agonist
- *agonist-antagonists*: drugs that are agonists at one opioid receptor type and antagonists at another

SIDE EFFECTS OF OPIOIDS

The opioids commonly used for pain management act primarily at μ receptor sites and therefore all have a similar spectrum of side effects (**Box 2.2**). In equianalgesic doses (doses that have the same analgesic effect) and in most patients, the incidence of side effects is generally very similar regardless of the opioid used.

Opioid receptors	
Receptor	Action
Mu (μ)	Analgesia, respiratory depression, euphoria, bradycardia, pruritus, miosis, nausea and vomiting, inhibition of gut motility
Kappa (κ)	Analgesia, sedation, miosis
Delta (δ)	Analgesia
Sigma (σ)	Psychotomimetic effects (e.g. dysphoria, hallucinations), mydriasis

Box 2.1

Possible side effects of opioids	
Respiratory	Respiratory depression
Central nervous system	Sedation, euphoria (sometimes dysphoria), nausea and vomiting, miosis, muscle rigidity
Cardiovascular	Vasodilatation, bradycardia, myocardial depression
Pruritus	More common with morphine
Genitourinary	Urinary retention
Gastrointestinal	Delayed gastric emptying, constipation, spasm of the sphincter of Oddi
Allergy	A true allergy is uncommon

Box 2.2

EFFECTS ON THE RESPIRATORY SYSTEM

Opioids can affect ventilatory pattern in a number of ways which may result in progressive clinical respiratory depression indicative of excessive opioid dose, or in episodes of intermittent hypoxemia which may develop with doses that are not excessive. The effects that can occur are:

- upper airway obstruction (obstructive apnea)
- a decrease in respiratory rate and/or changes in respiratory rhythm
- a decrease in tidal volume

With normal respiration, an increase in tone of the muscles of the upper airway precedes contraction of the diaphragm and inspiration. In the presence of opioids and sleep this coordination can be abolished and closure of the upper airway on inspiration may result. This may manifest itself as snoring (partial upper airway obstruction) or complete upper airway obstruction.

Opioids also directly depress the respiratory centre resulting in decreases in respiratory rate and tidal volume.

Respiratory depression

Respiratory depression is a relatively uncommon (though much-feared) complication of opioid administration. Traditionally respiratory rate has been used as an indicator of clinical respiratory depression, but a *decrease in respiratory rate is now recognized to be a late and unreliable sign.* A normal respiratory rate may coexist with marked respiratory depression. Because inadequate ventilation due to excessive doses of opioid can also result from upper airway obstruction or reductions in tidal volume (see above), the best clinical indicator of early respiratory depression is *sedation.* The sedation is presumed to be a combined effect of the opioid and the increase in P_{CO_2} level.

Sedation can be monitored using a sedation score (**Box 2.3**). Any dose of opioid should be adjusted to ensure that the sedation score remains below 2.

When respiratory rate is counted it should be the *unstimulated* rate, that is before the patient is roused. In general a rate of less than 8 per minute is considered to indicate respiratory depression, although as mentioned before, respiratory depression can coexist with a normal respiratory rate.

The administration of sedatives (including benzodiazepines, antihistamines and some antiemetics) will markedly increase the risk of respiratory depression and they should not routinely be given to patients receiving opioids. If sedatives are considered necessary, smaller than normal doses should be used in the first instance. As well as increasing the risk of respiratory depression, the addition of a sedative can make it impossible to give sufficient opioid to achieve patient comfort without causing excessive sedation.

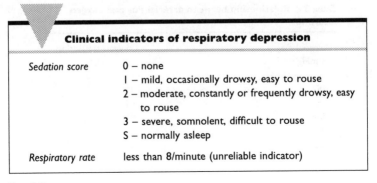

Clinical indicators of respiratory depression	
Sedation score	0 – none
	1 – mild, occasionally drowsy, easy to rouse
	2 – moderate, constantly or frequently drowsy, easy to rouse
	3 – severe, somnolent, difficult to rouse
	S – normally asleep
Respiratory rate	less than 8/minute (unreliable indicator)

Box 2.3

Changes in P_{O_2}, P_{CO_2} and oxygen saturation with respiratory depression Oxygen saturation, as measured by a pulse oximeter, is used in many wards as an easy and noninvasive measure of blood oxygen levels. However, care must be taken in the interpretation of any readings. If the patient is receiving supplemental oxygen, oxygen saturation may not be a good indicator of poor respiratory function, including respiratory depression. While low oxygen saturation levels in patients receiving oxygen indicate major abnormalities in respiratory function, normal oxygen saturation level, in patients receiving oxygen *do not* exclude abnormalities in respiratory function.

For example, a healthy young patient before an operation given oxygen at 4 litres per minute may have an arterial P_{O_2} of 130–150 mmHg. The pulse oximeter may show an oxygen saturation of 99%. The same patient after a major abdominal operation and receiving the same amount of oxygen may have a P_{O_2} of only 100 mmHg, but the oximeter will show only a small decrease in saturation to 98%; yet there is clearly some abnormality of lung function leading to a lesser than expected P_{O_2} for the inspired oxygen concentration. This would be even more obvious if a patient given oxygen at 10 l/min only had a P_{O_2} of 100 mmHg, far less than would be expected from this inspired oxygen concentration in normal lungs. The oxygen saturation would still be 98% despite obviously abnormal respiratory function.

The relationship between arterial P_{O_2} and oxygen saturation is

Table 2.1 Relationship between arterial P_{O_2} and oxygen saturation

Arterial P_{O_2} (mmHg)	Oxygen saturation (%)
100	98
90	97
80	95
70	93
60	90
40	75 (venous blood)
26	50

not linear, owing to the oxygen-hemoglobin dissociation curve (discussed in any physiology textbook). Some approximate values worth remembering are given in **Table 2.1**.

If arterial blood gas analysis shows an increased arterial P_{CO_2}, regardless of the P_{O_2} level, opioid-induced respiratory depression should be considered.

Pain antagonizes respiratory depression Pain is an effective antagonist to opioid-induced respiratory depression. If a patient has received a large dose of opioid as treatment for pain and then, for example, a local anesthetic block is given to manage that pain, onset of the block may be followed by respiratory depression. A similar result may follow if the cause of the pain is removed. For example, the opioids self-administered by a patient using PCA for the abdominal pain caused by urinary retention may cause respiratory depression when a urinary catheter is inserted and the pain settles.

All opioids in equianalgesic doses cause the same degree of respiratory depression. If opioids are properly titrated the risk of respiratory depression is small.

Intermittent episodes of hypoxemia

Hypoxemia can be caused by intermittent episodes of upper airway obstruction, as described above. The clinical picture is very similar to that seen in sleep apnea syndrome, and as in this syndrome, the intermittent airway obstruction and potentially profound decreases in oxygen saturation occur when the patient is asleep.

These episodes resembling sleep apnea can occur when opioids are being administered by any route and do not necessarily mean that excessive doses of opioid are being given. Arterial P_{CO_2} levels may remain within normal limits, and unless continuous pulse oximetry is being used, the episodes of hypoxemia are likely to be missed.

Hypoxemia, whether from these intermittent episodes of upper airway obstruction or from a progressive respiratory depression, can lead to tachycardia, arrhythmias, myocardial ischemia, confusion or short-term memory impairment, and possibly delayed wound healing. In an awake patient, hypoxemia is most often due to causes other than opioids.

Postoperative oxygen administration

Many patients will already have a background hypoxemia due to postoperative changes in lung function. Any episodes of apnea may therefore rapidly result in very low Po_2 levels. In addition, there is evidence to suggest that hypoxemia may be worse on about the third night after an operation. For these reasons, continuous oxygen administration for at least 2–3 days is sometimes recommended for patients given opioids after major operations, regardless of the route of administration of the opioid. Nasal cannulae with oxygen flows of 2–4 l/min will be adequate for most patients and are more likely to stay in place than a facemask. Supplemental oxygen will not affect the number of episodes of obstructive apnea but will reduce the severity of the subsequent falls in oxygen saturation levels.

EFFECTS ON THE CENTRAL NERVOUS SYSTEM

Nausea and vomiting

Opioids cause nausea and vomiting by stimulation of the chemoreceptor trigger zone in the medulla and the effects are enhanced by vestibular stimulation. Opioids also increase vestibular sensitivity. Even slight movement, such as turning the head, may be enough to trigger nausea and vomiting in some patients. For this reason, drugs that are used for motion sickness, such as transdermal scopolamine, are sometimes useful in the treatment of opioid-induced nausea and vomiting.

Opioids are not the only cause of postoperative nausea and vomiting (PONV). Other factors that have been shown to affect the incidence of PONV are patient age, gender, phase of menstrual cycle, anxiety, a full stomach, type and duration of surgery, history of motion sickness or previous PONV, anesthetic drugs and movement of the patient.

Opioid-related PONV is often dose-related and if the nausea and vomiting is thought to be due to the opioid, a trial of reduction in dose may be appropriate before a change to another opioid is made. Individual patients may be more sensitive to one particular opioid so changing to another opioid – e.g. from morphine to meperidine (pethidine) or hydromorphone – is worth considering if other measures have failed.

Miosis, sedation, euphoria and muscle rigidity
Opioids cause constriction of the pupils (miosis) and sedation, but it is important to remember that any sedation may indicate respiratory depression. While a mild euphoria may be associated with opioid administration, dysphoria and hallucinations occur occasionally. Muscle rigidity has been reported following doses of opioid larger than those normally used outside the operating room.

Confusion
Postoperative confusion is often blamed on opioids, but opioids in therapeutic doses are usually not the cause, or at least not the sole cause. A common and often easily reversible reason for postoperative confusion is hypoxia and this should be ruled out in all cases. Other causes of confusion include sleep deprivation, withdrawal from alcohol or other drugs, and sepsis. Elderly patients may become confused when placed in an unfamiliar environment.

EFFECTS ON THE CARDIOVASCULAR SYSTEM
Opioids cause arterial and venous vasodilatation by a direct effect on vascular smooth muscle. Some opioids, notably morphine, diamorphine, meperidine and codeine, may release histamine which will also lead to vasodilatation. Postural (orthostatic) hypotension may occur when a supine patient sits or stands. If a significant decrease in blood pressure is seen following administration of an opioid in a supine patient, it is often because the patient is also hypovolemic.

Opioids can also produce a vagally mediated bradycardia. The exception is meperidine, which may cause a slight tachycardia due to its atropine-like effects.

PRURITUS

Some opioids cause histamine release from mast cells which may result in local or generalized itching. If these opioids are given by intravenous injection, a localized urticaria may sometimes be seen at the site of injection or along the track of the vein into which the drug is being injected. This is due to local histamine release and does not usually indicate a true allergy to the opioid.

Although the exact mechanism of action is not known, pruritus due to opioids may also be centrally mediated, presumed to be a consequence of μ receptor activation. It is not associated with a rash and is not an allergic response to the drug. It is more common following epidural or intrathecal administration of opioids.

Pruritus is more common with morphine than with meperidine or fentanyl and does not always require treatment. If the patient is disturbed by this side effect, the safest treatment in the first instance is to change drugs. Antihistamines, because of their sedative effects, may add to the risk of sedation and respiratory depression. The pruritus may also respond to small, carefully titrated doses of intravenous naloxone. There is a risk that naloxone may also reverse some of the analgesic effects of the opioid, although this is less likely if the pruritus follows the administration of an epidural or intrathecal opioid. Intravenous nalbuphine, in small doses, is also effective in some cases.

EFFECTS ON THE GASTROINTESTINAL AND GENITOURINARY SYSTEMS

Opioids alter smooth muscle activity leading to delayed gastric emptying, inhibition of bowel motility and constipation. This inhibition is both locally and centrally mediated. While some decrease in bowel motility is inevitable, it is usually not necessary or appropriate to withhold opioids to facilitate the return of bowel function after surgery.

Opioid agonists may also cause increases in biliary tract pressure and spasm of the sphincter of Oddi, which can be reversed by the administration of naloxone.

Urinary retention can occur and may also be reversed by naloxone, especially if it follows epidural or intrathecal opioid administration. It is not necessary for all patients receiving epidural or intrathecal opioid analgesia to be catheterized or to remain catheterized.

ALLERGY

Patients and staff alike will often mistakenly report any adverse reaction to a drug as an allergy (e.g. nausea and vomiting following the administration of opioids; gastrointestinal upsets following the administration of antibiotics). True allergic reactions to opioids are mediated by the immune system and result in signs and symptoms that are similar to other allergic reactions including rash, urticaria, bronchoconstriction, angioneurotic edema and cardiovascular disturbances.

PREDICTORS OF OPIOID DOSE

Traditionally the dose of opioid prescribed for a patient was based – if indeed it was based on anything – on the weight of the patient. In fact there is no clinically significant correlation between patient weight and opioid requirement. The best clinical predictor of opioid dose is *patient age*. **Figure 2.1** shows the average intravenous PCA morphine requirements of 1010 opioid-naive patients in the first 24 hours after major surgery. The total amount of morphine used in 24 hours decreased significantly with increasing patient age. From **Figure 2.1** it can be seen that the average first 24-hour morphine requirements were 80 mg, 54 mg and 36 mg for patients aged 20 years, 45 years and 70 years respectively. If a straight line is drawn through points representing 80 mg, 55 mg and 30 mg for these age groups (and the difference from the original points is well within the differences due to interpatient variation in each age group), it can be seen that after the age of 20 years, first 24-hour morphine requirements decrease by about 1 mg for each additional year of age; or:

Average first 24-hour morphine requirements (mg) for patients over 20 years = 100 − (age in years)

Note the enormous variation (eightfold to tenfold) in dose

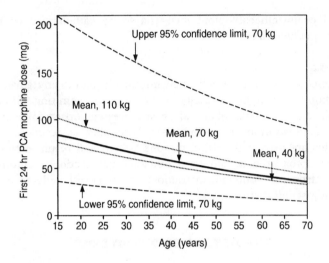

Figure 2.1
First 24-hour PCA morphine requirements and patient age. Adapted with permission from Macintyre and Jarvis (1995)

requirements in each age group. This means that although the initial dose of opioid should be based on the age of the patient, subsequent doses still need to be titrated to suit each patient.

Although the weight of the patient has some effect on dose, this is clinically insignificant in comparison to the overall interpatient variation.

There are a number of reasons why the dose of opioid required for pain relief should change with patient age: these include age-related alterations in the distribution of the drugs to different tissues, as well as in their metabolism and excretion. There may also be age-related changes in opioid receptor numbers or binding affinities.

TITRATION OF OPIOID DOSE

For an opioid to be effective it must reach a certain concentration in the blood (this applies to parenterally and enterally administered opioids, not to epidural and intrathecal opioids which are discussed in Chapter 6). The effective range of blood concentrations varies fourfold to fivefold between patients, and the amount of opioid that each patient requires will also vary according to the severity of the pain stimulus. Thus titration of opioids is needed to individualize treatment for each patient.

The lowest blood concentration of opioid that will produce analgesia is known as the *minimum effective analgesic concentration* (MEAC). Below this level a patient will experience no pain relief, and above it there will be increasing analgesia and an increasing possibility of side effects. In reality the boundaries are somewhat blurred and side effects may occur before good analgesia is obtained. The range of blood levels where analgesia is achieved without significant side effects is often colloquially referred to as the 'analgesic corridor' (**Figure 2.2**). For each patient the aim of

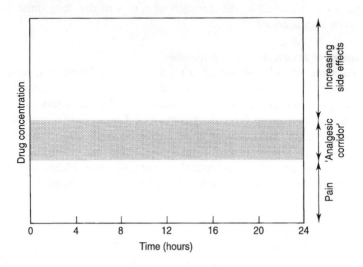

Figure 2.2
The 'analgesic corridor'

titration is to find and then maintain the effective blood level within this 'corridor'. A change in pain intensity may shift the 'corridor', requiring modification of opioid dose.

To enable opioid analgesia to be titrated to suit each patient, appropriate doses and dose intervals need to be ordered. In addition, endpoints that indicate adequate or excessive doses need to be monitored repeatedly.

DOSE RANGE
The range of doses prescribed should center around the average for the age of the patient and will vary according to the route of administration of the drug.

DOSE INTERVAL
When an interval is prescribed between intermittent doses of opioid, the aim of this interval is to allow the previous dose to have an effect before another dose is given, and to give some indication as to how long a single dose might be expected to exert an effect. Thus, the time taken for the drug to have its peak effect as well as the duration of action of the drug must be taken into account.

Onset of action and maximum effect
The time taken for an opioid to reach maximum blood concentration depends primarily on the route of administration. However, the time then taken to achieve maximum effect depends on the time it takes for the drug to cross the blood-brain barrier and bind to the opioid receptors in the central nervous system. Of the opioids in common clinical use, the least lipid-soluble, morphine, has the longest delay and it may take up to 15 minutes or more following intravenous injection for its maximum effect to be seen.

Duration of action
The duration of action of any given dose of opioid depends on a number of factors including the amount given, the route of administration and pharmacokinetic characteristics of the drug such as absorption, rate of distribution to different tissues

(including receptors), rate of dissociation from receptors and the elimination half-life $(t_{\frac{1}{2}\beta})$. The elimination half-life gives an indication of the time the body takes to metabolize and excrete the drug. It alone does not determine duration of action, it is only the time taken for the blood concentration of the drug to change by 50%. The drugs are metabolized to a form that is more easily excreted. In the case of opioids, the liver is the primary site of metabolism and the kidney the primary route of excretion of the metabolites. The metabolites of some of the opioids also have an analgesic action or additional undesirable actions.

MONITORING OF PAIN AND SEDATION SCORES AND OTHER SIDE EFFECTS

When titrating any drug, regular monitoring of endpoints that indicate 'how much is enough' and 'how much is too much' is needed. The best way to monitor the former is the pain score. The most serious consequence of excessive opioid dose is respiratory depression and, as outlined before, the best early indication of this is sedation, although respiratory rate is usually also counted. Nausea and vomiting or light-headedness may also indicate a slightly excessive dose.

The aim of pain treatment is to *make the patient comfortable while keeping the sedation score below 2*. If the patient does become sedated, subsequent doses should be reduced. If the patient is uncomfortable and not sedated, a larger dose is required (**Box 2.4**).

Some concurrent medical conditions or medications may affect

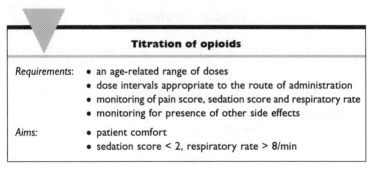

	Titration of opioids
Requirements:	• an age-related range of doses
	• dose intervals appropriate to the route of administration
	• monitoring of pain score, sedation score and respiratory rate
	• monitoring for presence of other side effects
Aims:	• patient comfort
	• sedation score < 2, respiratory rate > 8/min

Box 2.4

the metabolism or excretion of opioids and their metabolites. It is not possible to predict the degree of impairment from alterations in laboratory tests of renal or hepatic function, but careful titration will allow the appropriate adjustments in dose and dose interval to be made.

EQUIANALGESIC DOSES OF OPIOID DRUGS

All opioid agonists are capable of producing the same degree of pain relief and can be made equianalgesic if adjustments are made for dose and route of administration.

If a change is made from a parenteral (intramuscular, subcutaneous or intravenous) route to oral administration, larger doses will be needed because of the 'first pass' effect. That is, the proportion of an orally administered drug that is metabolized by the liver and gut wall after absorption from the gastrointestinal tract determines the amount of unchanged drug that reaches the systemic circulation.

The conversions listed in **Box 2.5** should be used as guidelines only.

Only drugs in common use are listed and not all will be available in every country. Formulations, generic names and trade names may vary.

OPIOID AGONISTS

The opioid agonist drugs are primarily μ receptor agonists.

MORPHINE
Morphine remains the standard against which all new analgesics are compared. Although newer analgesics may possess special qualities, none is clinically superior in relieving pain.

Morphine is the least lipid-soluble of all the opioids in common use. It is metabolized principally in the liver and the main metabolites are morphine 3-glucuronide, which has no analgesic

Equianalgesic doses

Opioid	IM/IV (mg)	Oral (mg)	$t_{1/2\beta}$ (hr)
Morphine	10	30–60	2–3
Meperidine (pethidine)	100	400	3–4
Papaveretum	15	(see morphine)	
Oxycodone	15	10–20	2–3
Codeine	130	200	3–4
Fentanyl	0.1	–	3–4
Diamorphine	5	60	0.5*
Methadone	10	20	15–40
Hydromorphone	1.5	7.5	2–3
Oxymorphone	1.0	–	2–3
Buprenorphine	0.4	0.8**	3–5
Pentazocine	40–60	150	3–5
Nalbuphine	10–20		3–6
Butorphanol	2		3

* rapidly hydrolysed to morphine
** sublingual
Table compiled from values obtained from listed references

Box 2.5

action, and morphine 6-glucuronide, which is approximately twice as potent an analgesic as morphine. The glucuronides are primarily excreted via the kidney, and renal impairment will lead to a build-up of these metabolites. Less than 10% of morphine is excreted unchanged by the kidneys. The half-life of morphine is not increased in patients with reduced renal function, although there may be an apparent prolongation of the effect of morphine. This is due to accumulation of morphine 6-glucuronide.

Morphine can be given by intramuscular, intravenous, subcutaneous, oral, rectal, epidural and intrathecal routes. Dose ranges and dose intervals will vary according to the route of administration.

Slow or sustained release preparations of oral morphine are available for the treatment of chronic and cancer pain and only need to be given two or three times a day. The slower onset and longer duration of action of the sustained release formulations make fast titration of the drug impossible, and these preparations are unsuitable for the treatment of acute pain.

MEPERIDINE (PETHIDINE)

Meperidine was first synthesized just prior to World War II as a potential substitute for atropine. In addition to its analgesic effect, meperidine has some atropine-like actions which may lead to a dry mouth or slight tachycardia, and some local anesthetic activity (this latter effect has allowed intrathecal meperidine, see Chapter 6, to be used as the sole agent for spinal anesthesia). Myocardial depression can occur with larger doses. In patients taking mono-amine oxidase inhibitors, hyperpyrexia, convulsions, coma and hypertension or hypotension have been reported following the administration of meperidine.

Meperidine can be given by intramuscular or intravenous injection or infusion (subcutaneous injections may be excessively painful) as well as by oral, rectal, epidural and intrathecal routes. Like morphine, the range of doses and dose durations required will vary according to the route of administration.

Unlike the other opioids, meperidine has been used to treat the shivering associated with volatile anesthetic agents, epidural/spinal anesthesia and chemotherapy. The usual initial dose is 25 mg IV.

Meperidine is primarily metabolized in the liver and the metabolites excreted by the kidney. Less than 10% of meperidine is excreted unchanged by the kidneys. One of the main metabolites is normeperidine (norpethidine) which has a long half-life ($t_{\frac{1}{2}\beta}$) of 15–20 hours. Unlike the other opioids, a build-up of this metabolite can cause signs and symptoms of central nervous system excitation, called normeperidine toxicity.

Normeperidine (norpethidine) toxicity

Normeperidine is a μ agonist and is therefore analgesic, but it has other nonopioid effects on the central nervous system (CNS). High blood levels can lead to anxiety, mood change, tremors, twitching, myoclonic jerks and even frank convulsions (**Box**

2.6). Patients receiving large doses of meperidine or those with renal impairment are particularly at risk.

Signs of normeperidine toxicity can be seen within 24–36 hours in some healthy patients with normal renal function requiring doses in the higher range for each age group. It was probably not seen in this group of patients until recently because very few patients would have been given more than 100 mg meperidine 4-hourly – a total of only 600 mg a day. With the advent of patient-controlled analgesia (PCA) patients can receive much higher doses, and therefore normeperidine levels may rise more rapidly.

There is no specific treatment for normeperidine toxicity. Meperidine should be discontinued and another opioid substituted. Naloxone should not be given as it will antagonize any sedative effect of meperidine but not the excitatory effects of normeperidine, and therefore will only exacerbate the problem.

As there is no specific treatment it is important to watch for early signs and symptoms of toxicity and prevent excessive levels of normeperidine by limiting the amount of meperidine administered. It is difficult to predict exactly what dose of meperidine or

Normeperidine (norpethidine) toxicity	
Effects of normeperidine	analgesia (μ receptor mediated)
	CNS excitation (nonopioid effect)
	$t_{1/2\beta}$: 15–20 hours
Signs and symptoms	anxiety, agitation, mood change, tremors, twitching, myoclonic jerks, convulsions
Treatment	• discontinue meperidine
	• substitute an alternative opioid
	• symptomatic treatment of effects
	• wait!
	DO NOT administer naloxone
Dose limits suggested	• 1000 mg in first 24 hours
	• 600–700 mg/day thereafter
	• these limits should be reduced in elderly patient or patients with renal impairment

Box 2.6

what blood level of normeperidine is likely to cause toxicity in any particular patient. However, it is suggested that the young patient with normal renal function should not receive more than 1000 mg in the first 24 hours of treatment. Subsequent totals should probably not exceed 600–700 mg per 24 hours. These limits should be reduced for elderly patients and patients with renal impairment.

PAPAVERETUM

Like opium, papaveretum contains a mixture of alkaloids. The percentage of morphine by weight is 50%. Although it is a popular choice of drug in Britain and Australia, there is no advantage in using this preparation compared with using morphine alone.

OXYCODONE

Oxycodone is a thebaine derivative. It can be given by parenteral, oral and rectal routes. Because oxycodone was first introduced into some countries in oral formulations combined with acetaminophen (paracetamol) or aspirin, it was considered suitable for the treatment of mild to moderate pain only. It is the limitations placed on the total dose of acetaminophen or aspirin that can be given to a patient in any one day that may limit the usefulness of the combined formulations. Alone and in higher doses, oxycodone can be used for the treatment of severe pain. Oxycodone is metabolized to noroxycodone.

CODEINE

Codeine is a naturally occurring alkaloid like morphine. It is metabolized in the liver where 5–10% of the dose is converted to morphine. This probably accounts for the main analgesic action of codeine, as the drug itself has a very low affinity for opioid receptors. Codeine is usually given for the treatment of mild to moderate pain by the intramuscular or oral route. Oral formulations that combine codeine with nonopioid analgesic drugs such as acetaminophen are often used.

FENTANYL

Fentanyl is a highly lipid-soluble synthetic opioid that does not cause histamine release. It has a more rapid onset of action than morphine and single doses have a short duration of action because of rapid tissue uptake. It is most frequently used as an intraoperative analgesic. The metabolites are inactive. For the treatment of acute pain it can be administered intravenously (for example, by patient-controlled analgesia pump), epidurally or intrathecally. Oral transmucosal administration has been used in children. Recently developed transdermal delivery systems for fentanyl have not proved universally successful for the management of acute pain. Onset of analgesia is slow, and residual drug depots in skin tissue may lead to sustained effects long after the patch has been removed.

DIAMORPHINE (HEROIN)

Diamorphine does not bind to opioid receptors and has no analgesic activity. It is a prodrug and is rapidly hydrolysed to 6-monoacetylmorphine (which has analgesic activity) and then morphine. It has not been shown to have any clinical advantage over morphine when administered by the oral or intramuscular route. Both diamorphine and 6-monoacetylmorphine are more lipid-soluble than morphine and cross the blood-brain barrier more rapidly; diamorphine therefore has a more rapid onset of action than morphine when given by the intravenous or epidural route. Diamorphine is not available for medical use in the USA or Australia.

METHADONE

A synthetic opioid developed during World War II, methadone has a much longer half-life and therefore a much longer duration of action than other opioids. This may make fast titration of methadone in the immediate postoperative period more difficult than using drugs with shorter half-lives. Methadone is more commonly used for the management of chronic pain or in drug dependency treatment programs. It can be given by oral, intravenous, intramuscular and epidural routes.

HYDROMORPHONE

A direct derivative of morphine, hydromorphone is available in oral, parenteral and suppository forms and can also be used for epidural analgesia. It has no active metabolites.

OXYMORPHONE

More lipid-soluble than morphine, oxymorphone is available in parenteral and suppository preparations.

OTHER OPIOIDS

The opioids listed below are commonly available as an oral formulation combined with a nonopioid analgesic, which limits the amount of the opioid that can be given.

Propoxyphene (dextropropoxyphene)

Structurally similar to methadone, only the dextrorotatory form has any analgesic activity (dextropropoxyphene). Often administered in an oral formulation in combination with acetaminophen (paracetamol) or aspirin, these preparations are probably only a little more effective than acetaminophen or aspirin alone. Toxicity, with hallucinations, delusions and confusion, may occur with accumulation of the renally excreted active metabolite norpropoxyphene, but this is unlikely to be significant at doses used clinically. The $t_{\frac{1}{2}\beta}$ is 6–12 hours.

Hydrocodone

Hydrocodone is available in the USA only in combination formulations with nonopioid analgesics such as acetaminophen. Its $t_{\frac{1}{2}\beta}$ is similar to codeine.

PARTIAL AGONISTS AND AGONIST-ANTAGONISTS

Buprenorphine is usually classed as a partial agonist and the other drugs listed below as agonist-antagonists. Agonist-antagonist drugs derive their analgesic actions principally from κ receptor activation while acting as antagonists at the μ receptor. Most of these drugs also at least partially activate the σ receptor. When given in doses that are equianalgesic to morphine these drugs result in the same side effects, although (unlike pure agonists), there is a ceiling effect for both analgesia and respiratory depression. The agonist-antagonist opioids are associated with a higher incidence of psychotomimetic effects (such as dysphoria) and sedation than pure agonist opioids.

These drugs are said to have a lower potential for abuse than other opioids, but this is of limited significance in patients with no previous history of substance abuse and in whom the risk of addiction to opioids used for the treatment of acute pain is minimal. The agonist-antagonist drugs can precipitate withdrawal signs and symptoms in opioid dependent patients.

On the whole, partial agonist and agonist-antagonist opioid drugs are used far less commonly in clinical practice than the pure opioid agonist drugs.

BUPRENORPHINE
Buprenorphine is derived from the opium alkaloid thebaine and is available in parenteral and sublingual formulations. It is highly lipid-soluble, hence its excellent absorption by the sublingual route. It dissociates very slowly from the μ receptor and therefore has a prolonged duration of action. Dysphoric side effects are relatively uncommon and other side effects are similar to morphine.

PENTAZOCINE
Pentazocine was the first drug of this class to become established in clinical practice. It can be given orally or parenterally. The high incidence of dysphoria associated with the drug has limited its continued use.

NALBUPHINE
Chemically related to naloxone, nalbuphine is available as an injectable preparation. It may be effective in reversing some of the side effects of μ agonist drugs, such as respiratory depression and pruritus.

BUTORPHANOL

Butorphanol is only available as a parenteral preparation.

OPIOID ANTAGONISTS

The opioid antagonists act at all receptor sites. The most commonly used of these drugs is naloxone.

NALOXONE

The $t_{\frac{1}{2}\beta}$ of naloxone, about 60 minutes, is much shorter than that of the drugs listed above. As a result, if naloxone is required to antagonize the effects of these drugs, repeated doses or an infusion may be needed. By titrating the dose of naloxone, it is possible to reverse opioid-induced respiratory depression and excessive sedation while still retaining reasonable analgesia. Small doses of naloxone can also be given to treat pruritus and urinary retention associated with opioid administration – see previous section on side effects of opioids.

The initial dose is 40–100 µg given intravenously and repeated every few minutes as required. If, for any reason, there is no venous access available, naloxone can be given in larger doses (e.g. 400 µg) by subcutaneous or intramuscular injection. If a patient is on chronic opioid therapy, it is especially important to titrate the doses of naloxone to avoid precipitation of withdrawal signs and symptoms.

While some cardiovascular stimulation (hypertension, tachycardia) or nausea and vomiting may be seen after administration of naloxone, especially after rapid reversal of analgesia, serious side effects such as pulmonary edema and arrhythmias are rare.

OPIOID TOLERANCE, DEPENDENCE AND ADDICTION

A major concern for both staff and patients is the fear of addiction to opioids given to relieve pain and this has led to undertreatment of pain in many instances. In fact, the risk of addiction from opioids taken to relieve acute pain is very small. In 11 882 inpatients given at least one opioid preparation, Porter and Jick (1980) noted that there were only four documented cases of addiction in patients with no prior history of substance abuse – an incidence of 0.03%. It has been said that those who prescribe and administer the opioids are more at risk of addiction than the patients receiving them.

Occasionally, staff may report that a patient is 'becoming addicted' to opioids when dose requirements seem to be higher than 'normal' or when the patient appears to be demanding pain-relieving drugs. Patients may seek or demand more analgesia if pain relief is inadequate. Undertreatment of pain may lead to a drug-seeking behavior which is really a pain-avoidance behavior and has been termed *pseudoaddiction* by Weisman and Heddox (1989).

Addiction to opioids must be distinguished from tolerance and from physical dependence on opioids (**Box 2.7**). All patients, whether addicted to opioids or receiving opioids for the treatment of pain over a prolonged period, will develop *physical dependence* and may show signs and symptoms of opioid withdrawal (abstinence syndrome) if the drug is antagonized, suddenly stopped, or markedly reduced in dose. Patients with an addiction to opioids will also have a *psychological dependence* on the drug which will be associated with drug-seeking behaviors.

Patients given high doses of opioids for as little as 7–10 days may show some signs of withdrawal if opioids are ceased abruptly. However, in most instances of treatment of acute pain, progressively less opioid is needed as the pain decreases. Withdrawal signs and symptoms can be prevented by daily tapered dose reductions of 20–25%.

Both groups of patients may also show a *tolerance* to opioids and need progressively larger doses to obtain the same analgesic effect.

A tolerance to the respiratory depressant effects of opioids also develops.

WITHDRAWAL (ABSTINENCE) SYNDROME

Signs and symptoms include yawning, sweating, lacrimation, rhinorrhea, anxiety, dilated pupils, piloerection, chills, tachycardia, hypertension, nausea and vomiting, crampy abdominal pains and diarrhea. Piloerection results in the appearance of gooseflesh so that the skin resembles that of a plucked turkey. Thus the expression 'cold turkey' is used to describe the syndrome of abrupt withdrawal from opioids.

▼ Opioid tolerance, dependence and addiction: definitions

Tolerance	A decrease in sensitivity to opioids so that progressively larger doses are needed to obtain the same analgesic effect.
Physical dependence	A physiologic state of adaptation to a drug usually characterized by the development of tolerance to the drug's effect and the emergence of a withdrawal (abstinence) syndrome if the drug is abruptly ceased or antagonized.
Psychological dependence	The emotional state of craving a drug either for its positive effect or to avoid negative effects associated with its absence.
Addiction	A chronic disorder characterized by the compulsive use of a substance resulting in physical, psychologic or social harm to the user and continued use despite that harm. There is a combination of a physical and psychological need for the drug associated with drug-seeking behaviors.
Pseudoaddiction	Drug-seeking behavior caused by a need for better pain relief

Adapted from Silverstein et al (1993)

Box 2.7

REFERENCES AND FURTHER READING

Benedetti C. (1990) Acute pain: a review of its effect and therapy with systemic opioids. In *Advances in Pain Research and Therapy* (Volume 14): *Opioid Analgesia* (eds Benedetti C., Chapman C.R. and Giron G.). Raven Press, New York.

Benedetti C. and Premuda L. (1990) The history of opium and its derivatives. In *Advances in Pain Research and Therapy* (Volume 14): *Opioid Analgesia* (eds Benedetti C., Chapman C.R. and Giron G.). Raven Press, New York.

Carr D.B., Jacox A.K., Chapman C.R. et al. (1992) *Acute Pain Management: Operative or Medical Procedures and Trauma, Clinical Practice Guideline.* AHCPR Pub. No. 92–0032. Rockville, MD: Agency for Health Care Policy and Research, Public Health Service, US Department of Health and Human Services.

Ferrante F.M. (1993) Opioids. In *Postoperative Pain Management* (eds Ferrante F.M. and VadeBoncouer T.R.). Churchill Livingstone, New York.

Jaffe J.H. (1992) Drug addiction and drug abuse. In *Goodman and Gilman's The Pharmacological Basis of Therapeutics* (eds Gilman A.J., Rall T.W., Nies A.J. and Taylor P.). McGraw-Hill International, Singapore.

Jaffe J.H. and Martin W.R. (1992) Opioid analgesics and antagonists. In *Goodman and Gilman's The Pharmacological Basis of Therapeutics* (eds Gilman A.J., Rall T.W., Nies A.J. and Taylor P.). McGraw-Hill International, Singapore.

Jones J.G., Sapsford D.J. and Wheatley R.G. (1990) Postoperative hypoxia: mechanisms and time course. *Anaesthesia* **45**, 566–573.

Kaiko R.F., Foley K.M., Grabinski P.Y., Heidrich G., Rogers A.G., Inturrisi C.E. and Reidenberg M.M. (1983) Central nervous system excitatory effects of meperidine in cancer patients. *Annals of Neurology* **13**, 180–185.

Macintyre P.E. and Jarvis D.A. (1995) Age is the best predictor of postoperative morphine requirements. *Pain* (in press).

Porter J. and Jick H. (1980) Addiction rare in patients treated with narcotics. *New England Journal of Medicine* **302**, 123.

Pöyhiä R., Vainio A. and Kalso E. (1993) A review of oxycodone's clinical pharmacokinetics and pharmacodynamics. *Journal of Pain and Symptom Management* **8**, 63–67.

Silverstein J.H., Silva D.A. and Iberti T.J. (1993) Opioid addiction in anesthesiology. *Anesthesiology* **79**, 354–371.

Stone P.A., Macintyre P.E. and Jarvis D.A. (1993) Norpethidine toxicity and patient-controlled analgesia. *British Journal of Anaesthesia* **71**, 738–740.

Watcha M.F. and White P.F. (1992) Postoperative nausea and vomiting. *Anesthesiology* **77**, 162–184.

Weisman D.E. and Heddox J.D. (1989) Opioid pseudoaddiction: an iatrogenic syndrome. *Pain* **36**, 363–366.

CHAPTER 3

PHARMACOLOGY OF LOCAL ANESTHETIC DRUGS

Mechanism of action;
Adverse effects of local anesthetic drugs;
Classes of local anesthetic drugs;
Commonly used local anesthetic drugs;
Equieffective anesthetic concentrations

The central stimulant effects of cocaine, obtained by chewing the leaves of the plant *Erythroxylon coca*, have been known for hundreds of years. Cocaine, an alkaloid contained in this plant (0.6–1.8% by weight), was first isolated in 1860 by Niemann, just a little over 50 years after morphine was first isolated from opium.

Cocaine was first introduced into medical practice in 1884 by Koller, who described its use for topical anesthesia of the cornea. This demonstration of the local anesthetic effect of cocaine was followed by its use for nerve conduction blockade and local infiltration anesthesia. In 1899 Bier reported on the use of cocaine for spinal anesthesia. By allowing himself to be the subject of one of his experiments, he demonstrated not only the effectiveness of this anesthetic technique but also that a severe postural headache could follow the introduction of a needle into cerebrospinal fluid.

Cocaine was also used in patent medicines. In 1886 Pemberton patented Coca Cola, a cola-flavored remedy. It was not until 1906 that the cocaine was replaced by caffeine and the product marketed as a soft drink.

The toxicity of cocaine and its brief duration of action limited its usefulness in surgical practice and led to a search for less toxic substances. The syntheses of prilocaine by Einhorn in 1905 and lidocaine (lignocaine) by Löfgren and Lundqvist in 1943 heralded the start of the further development of the local anesthetic drugs in common use today.

Until the 1980s the use of local anesthetic drugs was confined mainly to the immediate perioperative period. Since then, their use for acute pain management, either alone or in combination with opioids, and their administration on general surgical wards, has become increasingly popular and widespread.

MECHANISM OF ACTION

The generation and propagation of a nerve impulse along a nerve fiber involves the opening of sodium channels in the nerve membrane and the massive flow of sodium ions from the outside to the inside of the membrane. The local anesthetic drugs in common use act primarily by binding to receptor sites in the sodium channel, preventing this influx of sodium ions and thereby blocking conduction of the nerve impulse.

To do this the local anesthetic agent must first cross the cell membrane. Local anesthetic drugs exist in solution in two forms: a lipid-soluble (unionized) *base* and a water-soluble (ionized) *cationic* form. It is the lipid-soluble base that easily crosses the nerve membrane, and the water-soluble cationic form that blocks the sodium channel from the inside of the nerve membrane by attaching to a sodium channel binding site. If the tissues into which the local anesthetic agent is injected are more acid than normal (that is, the pH is lower than normal), as will happen if the tissues are infected, there is a decrease in the amount of the lipid-soluble base that is available to cross the nerve membrane, leading to a reduction in the effectiveness of the drug.

There are a number of different types of nerve fibers which vary in size and function (**Box 3.1**).

The ease with which a nerve fiber is blocked by a given concentration of local anesthetic drug depends on its *critical blocking length* (the length that must be exposed to the drug in order for the nerve to become blocked) and on the *accessibility* of the nerve membrane binding site to the blocking agent. It has always been

Nerve fiber class, size and function

Class	Size	Function
A-alpha (Aα)	Largest	Motor, proprioception (position sense)
A-beta (Aβ)		Touch/pressure, motor
A-gamma (Aγ)		Muscle spindle tone
A-delta (Aδ)		Pain/temperature
B		Preganglionic autonomic (sympathetic)
C (unmyelinated)	Smallest	Pain/temperature

Box 3.1

taught that smaller diameter nerve fibers are more easily blocked than larger diameter fibers. In fact, the actual diameter of the fiber is not itself important. However, the smaller diameter fibers have the smallest critical blocking length and are more easily accessed and blocked by local anesthetic solutions. Nerve blockade is also *frequency dependent*; that is, active nerve fibers are more easily blocked than inactive ones.

The onset and regression of a peripheral nerve block usually progresses according to the order in **Box 3.2**, but this may vary a little between patients and between the different drugs. Note that B fibers tend to be blocked before C fibers. This is probably because C fibers are usually arranged in Remak bundles, which

Onset and recovery of nerve block according to fiber class

	Order of onset	Order of recovery
first	B	Aα
	C, Aδ	Aβ
	Aγ	Aγ
	Aβ	Aδ, C
last	Aα	B

Box 3.2

may hamper diffusion of the local anesthetic solution, and/or because the critical blocking length of B fibers is quite short.

As the effect of any nerve block wears off, recovery of movement may precede recovery of sensation or sympathetic nerve function. This is of particular importance following epidural or spinal anesthesia, when a patient may appear to have normal motor function yet may have incomplete return of sensation and a residual sympathetic block that leads to postural (orthostatic) hypotension.

Epidural analgesia is increasing in popularity as a method of postoperative pain relief. Low concentrations of local anesthetic drugs are often used, usually mixed with opioids, in an attempt to preferentially block the smaller nerve fibers while avoiding a block of the large motor fibers (*differential nerve block*). This means that the patient may be able to move and walk normally while still receiving good pain relief. However, this cannot be assumed even if only low doses are being administered, and every patient should be assessed before ambulation is allowed. Note that while there is analgesia, blockade of sympathetic nerve fibers may be present and postural (orthostatic) hypotension remains a potential risk.

ADVERSE EFFECTS OF LOCAL ANESTHETIC DRUGS

The adverse effects that may follow the administration of a local anesthetic solution can be a result of the physiological effects of the nerves blocked, local tissue toxicity or systemic toxicity.

PHYSIOLOGICAL EFFECTS
Physiological effects are most common following epidural and spinal anesthesia or analgesia, and are covered in Chapter 6.

LOCAL TISSUE TOXICITY
The local anesthetic agents in common clinical use rarely produce localized nerve damage. Motor and sensory nerve deficits following subarachnoid administration of chloroprocaine were reported, probably due to the presence of the antioxidant, sodium bisul-

phite, in the solution. The sodium bisulphite was replaced with ethylenediaminetetraacetate (EDTA) in later formulations. More recently neurotoxicity has been reported following the administration of hyperbaric 5% lidocaine solutions, given by single injection or via microspinal catheters.

SYSTEMIC TOXICITY

High blood concentrations of the drugs may lead to signs and symptoms of systemic local anesthetic toxicity. This can occur if excessive doses of local anesthetic agents are given, or if an otherwise safe dose is inadvertently injected directly into a blood vessel. The higher the blood concentration of the local anesthetic drug, the more severe the signs and symptoms of toxicity.

A number of factors will influence the blood concentrations of local anesthetic drug reached after injection:

- *dose of drug*: this should be appropriate for the patient and the local block procedure employed. 'Recommended' or 'safe' doses may be overdoses if injected directly into blood vessels or tissues with a rich vascular supply
- *site of injection*: the rate of absorption of local anesthetic agents depends to a large extent on the blood supply to the area. The order from most to least rapid is: interpleural > intercostal > caudal > epidural > brachial plexus > subcutaneous infiltration
- *vasoconstrictor*: with some local anesthetic drugs (short to medium duration) the addition of a vasoconstrictor such as epinephrine (adrenaline) will decrease the rate of absorption of the drug into the circulation
- *speed of injection*: the more rapid the rate of injection the more rapid the rise in plasma concentration of the drug. In a general ward a continuous infusion of local anesthetic solution is the safest method of administration
- *metabolism of the drug*

The systemic toxicity of local anesthetic drugs results from their effects on the central nervous system (CNS) and cardiovascular system (**Box 3.3**). Not all of the signs and symptoms listed will necessarily occur in every patient.

**Signs and symptoms of systemic
local anesthetic toxicity**

Cardiovascular depression
Respiratory arrest
Coma
Convulsions
Drowsiness   *Increasing blood concentrations*
Muscular twitching
Tinnitus, visual disturbances
Circumoral numbness and
    numbness of tongue
Light-headedness

Box 3.3

Central nervous system toxicity

Signs and symptoms of CNS toxicity are generally seen at lower blood concentrations than those leading to cardiovascular toxicity. The early signs of CNS toxicity are those of CNS excitation and this is due to initial blockade of inhibitory pathways. Early signs are best detected by talking to the patient who, as blood concentrations of the drug rise, may complain of numbness around the mouth and tongue, a feeling of light-headedness and ringing in the ears. Slurring of the speech and muscle twitching will follow and the patient may become drowsy. If the blood level continues to rise a generalized convulsion (usually brief) will occur, and at even higher blood concentrations respiratory depression and arrest will ensue.

Hypercarbia and acidosis decrease the convulsive threshold of the drug increasing the risk of convulsions at lower blood levels. Conversely, hyperventilation will lower $P\text{CO}_2$ levels and help raise the seizure threshold, shortening the duration of the seizure. Hypoxia also enhances local anesthetic CNS toxicity.

If the patient has a generalized convulsion the main aims of treatment are to prevent cerebral and myocardial hypoxia, so oxygenation and ventilation are the first priorities. Small doses of an anticonvulsant such as midazolam, diazepam or (administered by anesthesia staff only) thiopental (thiopentone), should be given intravenously. Intubation of the patient may be necessary if ventilation is difficult, the patient is apneic or there is a need to protect the airway.

Cardiovascular toxicity
It is traditionally taught that cardiovascular toxicity normally only occurs at blood concentrations higher than those that result in signs of CNS toxicity. However, with bupivacaine and etidocaine, life-threatening arrhythmias or asystole have preceded convulsions, occurring with little or no warning.

Local anesthetic drugs can directly affect the muscles of the heart and peripheral blood vessels, and toxicity may result in alterations to myocardial contractility, conductivity and rhythmicity. Acidosis, hypercarbia and hypoxia markedly enhance the cardiotoxicity of local anesthetic drugs; it is therefore vital to treat any convulsion promptly and effectively.

Classes of local anesthetic drugs

Amides	Esters
Lidocaine (lignocaine)	Procaine
Bupivacaine	Chloroprocaine
Prilocaine	Cocaine
Dibucaine (cinchocaine)	Tetracaine
Mepivacaine	Benzocaine
Etidocaine	
Ropivacaine	

Box 3.4

CLASSES OF LOCAL ANESTHETIC DRUGS

Local anesthetic agents are classified according to the nature of the linkage between the lipid-soluble and water-soluble parts of the molecule. The two types of linkage are *amide* and *ester* (**Box 3.4**). The clinical differences between the two classes involve:

- the mechanisms by which they are metabolized
- their potential for producing allergic reactions

AMIDES

Amide local anesthetic drugs are metabolized in the liver, and the elimination half-lives vary from about 1.5 hours to 3.5 hours. These drugs rarely cause allergic reactions, although patients may be allergic to preservatives contained in some local anesthetic solutions. Some patients reporting an 'allergy' to these drugs may have experienced effects due to the systemic absorption of epinephrine or had a vasovagal response to the injection.

ESTERS

Ester local anesthetic drugs are metabolized in plasma by pseudocholinesterases, thus their half-lives in the circulation are shorter than the amides. Ester local anesthetic drugs have a higher incidence of allergic reactions.

COMMONLY USED LOCAL ANESTHETIC DRUGS

AMIDES

Bupivacaine

Bupivacaine is long-acting and is the most common local anesthetic agent in use for the management of acute pain outside the operating room. When used in the ward setting, low doses and administration by infusion will minimize the risk of toxicity. Bupivacaine is potentially more cardiotoxic than the other local anesthetic drugs and any cardiovascular collapse that does occur may be more difficult to treat. The addition of epinephrine (adrenaline) has little effect on the duration of action of the drug. One of the appealing features of bupivacaine is its high sensory block to motor block ratio, i.e. good analgesia can be obtained while motor function is retained.

Ropivacaine

Of a similar structure and potency to bupivacaine, ropivacaine is a newer local anesthetic agent which has a similar onset and duration of action to bupivacaine but is less cardiotoxic. In concentrations producing comparable analgesia, it results in less motor blockade than bupivacaine.

Lidocaine (lignocaine)

Lidocaine has a shorter duration of action than bupivacaine, although duration of action can be increased by the addition of epinephrine to the solution. Although widely used in regional and local anesthesia for operative procedures, it is not in common use for the ward management of acute pain. Lidocaine is available in a number of preparations: ointments, jelly, topical solutions including a spray, and formulations for injection. It has also been administered by nebulizer to obtain topical anesthesia of the upper airway. Intravenous lidocaine is used for the treatment of cardiac arrhythmias and some chronic pain states.

A mixture of lidocaine and prilocaine (2.5% of each), called EMLA^{TM} cream (eutectic mixture of local anesthetics), can be used as a topical local anesthetic agent for skin. Applied under an occlusive dressing or as a patch, it takes 30–60 minutes to have its full effect. It has been used prior to the insertion of intravenous cannulae or other needles (especially in children) and for local procedures such as superficial skin surgery, skin grafting and other minor surgery.

Mepivacaine

Mepivacaine has a similar anesthetic profile to lidocaine with a relatively rapid onset and a moderate duration of action.

Etidocaine

Etidocaine is as long-acting as bupivacaine and has been associated with similar problems with respect to cardiotoxicity. It is noted for its profound motor blockade.

Prilocaine

Prilocaine has a very similar clinical profile to lidocaine but is the least toxic of the amide local anesthetic drugs. This makes it a very suitable choice for intravenous regional anesthesia (Bier's block).

The initial step in the metabolism of prilocaine forms orthotoluidine and the administration of large doses of prilocaine may lead to the accumulation of this metabolite which, in turn, leads to an increase in the oxidation of hemoglobin to methemoglobin. If the level of methemoglobin reaches 3–5 mg/ml the patient may appear cyanotic.

Dibucaine (cinchocaine)

Dibucaine is used primarily for spinal anesthesia.

ESTERS

Cocaine

Cocaine has a number of actions in addition to its ability to block conduction of nerve impulses and produce local anesthesia. It causes a general stimulation of the CNS and blocks the reuptake of catecholamines at adrenergic nerve endings, thus potentiating the effects of sympathetic nervous system stimulation. These changes can lead to euphoria and a feeling of well-being, restlessness, excitement, tachycardia, peripheral vasoconstriction, hypertension, arrhythmias, myocardial ischemia and convulsions. Because of its relatively high potential for toxicity, cocaine is now restricted to use as a topical anesthetic agent, usually in surgery involving the nose or preceding nasal endotracheal intubation, where its local vasoconstrictor effect helps to shrink nasal mucosa and reduce bleeding. Doses should be kept within recommended limits to avoid risking the other side effects of cocaine.

Tetracaine

Like dibucaine, tetracaine is primarily used for spinal anesthesia.

Procaine

Procaine was the first synthetic local anesthetic introduced into clinical practice but its use is now confined mainly to local infiltration.

Chloroprocaine

Because of its rapid onset, rapid metabolism and short duration of action, chloroprocaine has been primarily used for obstetric epidural analgesia or regional anesthetic techniques for day surgery. Neurotoxicity with motor and sensory deficits has followed the accidental subarachnoid injection of this drug and the sodium bisulphite antioxidant in the anesthetic solution was implicated. In later formulations EDTA has replaced the bisulphite, but this has been followed by reports of muscle spasm and backache.

Equieffective anesthetic concentrations

Local anesthetic drug	Concentration (%)
Chloroprocaine	2
Tetracaine	0.25
Procaine	2
Cocaine	
Bupivacaine	0.25
Lidocaine (lignocaine)	1
Ropivacaine	0.25
Mepivacaine	1
Etidocaine	0.25
Prilocaine	1

Box 3.5

EQUIEFFECTIVE ANESTHETIC CONCENTRATIONS

Just as opioids have equianalgesic doses, if given in equal volumes local anesthetic drugs have equieffective anesthetic concentrations (**Box 3.5**).

REFERENCES AND FURTHER READING

Cousins M.J. (1993) Local anaesthetics and pain management. In *Advances in Pain Therapy II* (eds Chrubasik J., Cousins M. and Martin E.). Springer-Verlag, Berlin.

Covino B.G. (1993) Local anesthetics. In *Postoperative Pain Management* (eds Ferrante F.M. and VadeBoncouer T.R.) Churchill Livingstone, New York.

De Jong R.H. (1994) *Local Anesthetics.* Mosby, St Louis.

Denson D.D. and Mazoit J.X. (1992) Physiology and pharmacology of local anesthetics. In *Acute Pain – Mechanisms and Management* (eds Sinatra R.S., Hord A.H., Ginsberg B. and Preble L.M.). Mosby Year Book, St Louis.

Fink B.R. (1988) History of neural blockade. In *Neural Blockade in Clinical Anesthesia and Management of Pain* (eds Cousins M.J. and Bridenbaugh P.O.). J.B. Lippincott, Philadelphia.

Ritchie J.M. and Greene N.M. (1992) Local anesthetics. In *Goodman and Gilman's – The Pharmacological Basis of Therapeutics* (eds Gilman A.J., Rall T.W., Nies A.J. and Taylor P.). McGraw-Hill International, Singapore.

CHAPTER 4

TRADITIONAL METHODS OF OPIOID ADMINISTRATION

Intramuscular administration;

Intermittent subcutaneous administration;

Oral administration;

Intermittent intravenous administration;

Continuous intravenous infusions;

Continuous subcutaneous infusions;

Rectal administration

The introduction of more sophisticated methods for the administration of opioids, such as patient-controlled and epidural analgesia, has undoubtedly improved the management of acute pain. However, the more traditional and conventional methods of administration remain in common use, even in centers where the more advanced techniques are available. Numerous studies have shown that these methods have often not provided good analgesia, yet few attempts have been made to improve their effectiveness.

Lasagna and Beecher (1954) wrote that, for subcutaneous morphine, the 'optimal dose appears to be 10 mg per 70 kg of body weight'. That teaching has changed little over the intervening years. It makes no allowances for the enormous interpatient variation in opioid requirements (eightfold to tenfold) that result from the unpredictable differences in pharmacokinetic factors (how the individual patient handles the drug – i.e. how it is absorbed, distributed, metabolized and excreted) and pharmacodynamic factors (how the individual responds to the drug). The same dose of opioid given to different patients can result in a fourfold to fivefold difference in peak blood levels reached; the peak blood concentration from the same dose of opioid may vary twofold within the same patient; there is a fourfold to fivefold interpatient variation in the minimum effective analgesic concentration (MEAC). Added to this has been the lack of appropriate education of medical and nursing staff, resulting in an inadequate knowledge of the drugs they prescribe and administer and unfounded fears about the risks of side effects and addiction, and a lack of assessment of pain and the results (or otherwise) of its treatment. It is hardly surprising that standard regimens for pain relief have been less than successful.

The key to making these methods more effective is to individualize the opioid treatment regimen for each patient. Effectiveness of analgesia and possible side effects need to be monitored regularly and dose and frequency of administration altered accordingly so that each drug, regardless of route, is titrated to suit each patient. It is also important to allow the patient, where possible, some input into the size of the dose and the timing of each dose. 'Patient-controlled' should not be confined to patient-controlled analgesia (PCA) pump systems.

INTRAMUSCULAR ADMINISTRATION

Although morphine was first given by subcutaneous (SC) injection, the intramuscular (IM) route has become the more common route of administration, in the belief (somewhat mistaken) that absorption is slower from subcutaneous sites.

Traditionally, IM opioids have been ordered 4-hourly 'PRN' (*pro re nata* – meaning 'according to circumstances' or 'as the situation requires'). A reluctance to order or give opioids more frequently than this has played a major role in the lack of effectiveness of IM regimens. Even if pain returns before the end of this period, which is not uncommon, patients are often made to wait until the 4 hours has elapsed before they are 'allowed' another injection.

Figure 4.1 is a hypothetical representation of what could happen to the blood concentrations of a typical opioid with a half-life of

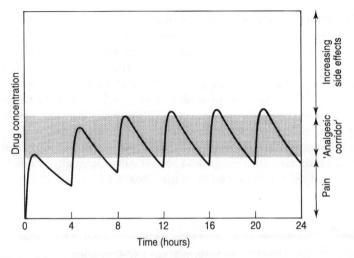

Figure 4.1
Intermittent intramuscular opioid analgesia

about 3 hours (e.g. morphine or meperidine) if the same IM dose is repeated at 4-hourly intervals.

After absorption from the injection site the first dose may result in a blood level that only just enters the 'analgesic corridor' for that patient, leading to very little if any pain relief. The second two doses may result in higher blood levels and better pain relief for longer periods. Fourth and subsequent doses may increase blood concentrations to a level that, as well as giving pain relief, starts to produce side effects.

Two things are obvious from Figure 4.1:

- the amount of opioid required to make a patient comfortable in the first instance is not the same as the amount required to maintain comfort
- while 'peaks and troughs' in the blood levels of opioid are an inevitable consequence of this type of regimen, the aim of treatment should be to reduce the extent of this variation so that the peaks and troughs occur predominantly within the 'analgesic corridor'. For example, giving a little less opioid more often can result in the same overall daily dose but less variability in blood concentrations between doses

TITRATION OF INTERMITTENT IM OPIOIDS

As outlined in Chapter 2, blood levels of an opioid need to reach the minimum effective analgesic concentration for each patient before any relief of pain is perceived. Furthermore, the effective range of blood levels varies some fourfold to fivefold between patients. The only way to achieve good pain relief is to titrate the dose of opioid for each patient. This requires the prescription of an appropriate initial dose and dose interval, followed by monitoring of the effectiveness of the analgesia and of signs that would indicate an excessive dose so that subsequent alterations to dose and dose interval can be made (**Box 4.1**).

Titration of intermittent IM/SC opioids

Requires:

An initial age-related range of morphine doses based on average daily requirement	Approximate average 24-hour morphine requirement for patients more than 20 years old = 100 − age (see Chapter 2)*
	single dose = average 24-hour morphine requirement ÷ 8
An appropriate dose interval	e.g. 2-hourly PRN or fixed interval
Monitoring of pain score, sedation score and respiratory rate	e.g. at time of injection and 1 hour after injection
Monitoring for presence of other side effects	
Selection of subsequent doses according to patient response	see Box 4.2

Aims for:

patient comfort, sedation score < 2 and respiratory rate > 8/min

*Taken from Figure 2.1, data refer to PCA morphine requirements in opioid-naive patients after major surgery and are approximations only. Variations may occur with different patient populations. These are *average* doses. The doses required by individual patients will vary widely.

Box 4.1

Dose range

As for any route, an age-related range of doses should be pre-scribed initially. A guide to total daily morphine doses can be obtained from **Figure 2.1** in Chapter 2 where it can be seen that the *approximate average 24-hour morphine requirements for patients over 20 years old = 100 − age*. Division of these 24-hour doses by 8 gives a reasonable indication of a value for the middle of an appropriate dose range for patients of a particular age. Although division by 8 assumes a 3-hourly dose, it is reasonable to add additional flexibility by ordering the range of doses 2-hourly PRN.

Note that these values were obtained from opioid-naive patients after major surgery. Variations may occur with different patient populations, and dose requirements may be less following minor surgery or for patients with pre-existing opioid usage.

Staff are often tempted to start at the lower limit of any pre-scribed range, but these ranges should allow them the ability to decrease as well as increase subsequent doses as required. Unless the clinical situation dictates it (e.g. the patient has severe pain or is a little sleepy) and provided the range ordered is appropriate, it is reasonable to start in the middle of the dose range in most cases.

Dose interval

The aims of a dose interval are to allow the previous dose to exert its effect before an additional dose is given, and provide an indication of how long a single dose may be expected to have an effect.

PRN dose regimens Prescription of opioids PRN have been the mainstay of acute pain management (albeit often inadequate management) for years. There are both drawbacks and advantages to the PRN system. It should mean that the opioid is given when the patient needs it; however, there are frequently long delays between the return of discomfort and the actual adminis-tration of more opioid. For a variety of reasons a patient may be reluctant to request another injection, at least until the pain is severe. In addition there are the inevitable delays that follow such a request in many hospitals, as opioids are kept in locked cup-boards and extra staff may be required to check the drug and dose before it is administered. Following administration there is yet another delay while the drug takes effect. Unless the patient is offered pain relief frequently, or asks for and is given another dose as soon as pain starts to become uncomfortable, the PRN system will fail.

The main advantage of a PRN regimen is that, titrated properly, it can provide the flexibility needed to cover the changes in pain stimulus that occur within each patient with acute pain.

With a PRN regimen, a dose interval really only has to ensure that a dose of opioid has had its maximum effect before another is given. For an intramuscular injection this means the time taken for the drug to be absorbed and reach a peak blood concentration plus the time taken to exert its maximum effect on the central nervous system. In most patients this would occur within an hour. Therefore, if a patient is in pain, there is no need to wait 4 hours before giving the next dose. A reasonable dose interval that allows for both safety and flexibility would be 2 hours. This does not mean that the drug has to be given every 2 hours but that it can be given if needed, although if a patient complains of pain within this time additional analgesia should not be withheld.

Fixed-interval dose regimens   Intramuscular opioids can also be given at fixed intervals. One reason for this approach being less popular than PRN regimens may be that opioid requirements vary enormously between patients and can be difficult to predict. In addition, especially after major injury or operation, the level of pain can fluctuate markedly within each patient according to different pain stimuli (physiotherapy or dressing changes, for example), as well as decrease a little each day. Fixed-interval dosing may not allow adequate flexibility and coverage of these episodes of 'incident' pain, or allow for the progressive reduction in dose requirements that will occur as the patient recovers. If fixed-interval regimens are used a range of doses should be available and the interval may need to be less than the traditional 4 hours. Additional PRN opioid orders may also be needed for breakthrough pain.

Monitoring

As outlined in Chapter 2, monitoring of pain scores, sedation scores and respiratory rates will give an indication of 'how much is enough' and 'how much is too much' opioid. For intermittent IM regimens, it would be reasonable to record these values when an injection is given (assuming it is given truly 'on demand') and 1 hour later, when the full effect of the injection can be seen. As with all opioids, the aim is to make the patient comfortable while keeping the sedation score less than 2 (see **Box 2.3**).

The onset of other opioid-related side effects, such as nausea and vomiting or pruritus, may be distressing to the patient. If nausea and vomiting appear to be related to the opioid (there are many causes of postoperative emesis), it may be reasonable to try smaller subsequent doses as well as administer an anti-emetic. Individual patients may be more sensitive to one particular opioid so changing to another opioid is worth considering if other measures have failed.

If the patient complains of pruritus it is worth trying a different opioid. Morphine in particular is associated with a higher incidence of itching than meperidine (pethidine) or fentanyl. As the pruritus is not necessarily due to histamine release, antihistamines may not be completely effective and, when administered with opioids, can increase the risk of respiratory depression. Intravenous nalbuphine (2.5–5 mg 4-hourly PRN) may be useful in some cases where other measures have been ineffective.

Selection of subsequent doses

Although the dose range ordered and the initial dose given should be based on the age of the patient, subsequent doses need to be titrated to suit each patient. All too often subsequent doses are chosen because 'that was the dose given before' and not on the basis of patient assessment. A suggested protocol for this titration is outlined in **Box 4.2**. Where possible, patients should be allowed some choice in the size and timing of subsequent doses. They can be instructed to ask for a larger dose if analgesia was inadequate or a smaller dose if they felt sleepy or nauseated.

• pethidine should NOT be given subcutaneously •

• for intermittent administration of intravenous opioids refer to appropriate RAH guidelines •

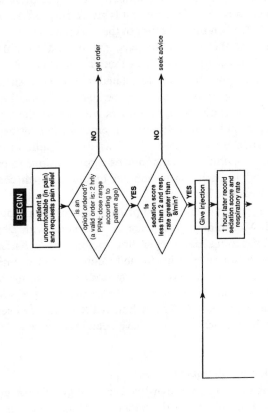

BEGIN

patient is uncomfortable (in pain) and requests pain relief

is an opioid ordered? (a valid order is : 2 hrly PRN; dose range according to patient age)

NO → get order

YES

Is sedation score less than 2 and resp. rate greater than 8/min?

NO → seek advice

YES

Give injection

1 hour later record sedation score and respiratory rate

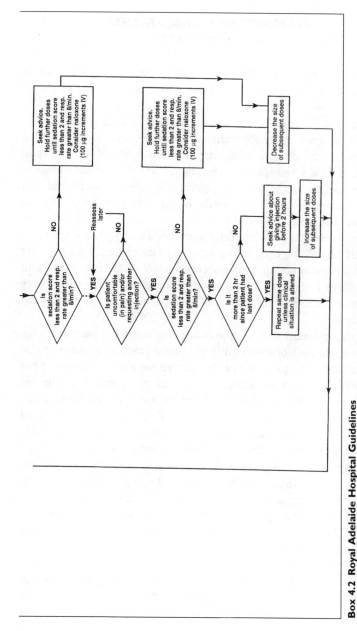

Box 4.2 Royal Adelaide Hospital Guidelines
INTERMITTENT SUBCUTANEOUS/INTRAMUSCULAR OPIOID ADMINISTRATION
for Acute Pain Management

INTERMITTENT SUBCUTANEOUS
ADMINISTRATION

The subcutaneous route is often used for opioid administration in the treatment of cancer pain; it can also be used in the treatment of acute pain.

An indwelling narrow-gauge butterfly needle or small IV cannula is inserted into subcutaneous tissue, for ease of access often just below the clavicle or the upper outer aspect of the arm, and covered with a transparent dressing. To ensure that the needle is placed correctly and not too superficially, a generous fold of skin and subcutaneous tissue should be held in one hand and the needle or cannula inserted at the base of this fold with the other. Injections are administered through a cap or one-way valve on the indwelling needle. Advantages of using this route over the IM route include improved patient comfort, as the number of skin punctures is decreased, and a reduced risk of needle stick injury as, once the indwelling needle is in place, all other needles can be avoided.

If the injection through the indwelling needle is painful it may be that the rate of injection is too rapid (each dose needs to be given over a few minutes) or that the needle has been inserted too superficially. The insertion site should be changed if pain on injection persists or if any redness or swelling develops at the site. Normally the indwelling needle will only need to be replaced every 3–4 days, although some institutions may require all indwelling cannulae to be changed at more frequent intervals.

Morphine is the drug most commonly used for intermittent subcutaneous (SC) injection. Meperidine (pethidine) tends to be too irritating and painful to be given by this route as a single injection (if the meperidine is diluted and given as an infusion or by PCA, irritation is not usually a problem). Subcutaneous opioids should be given in solutions concentrated enough to avoid the need for large volumes, as this can be another source of tissue irritation. As the rate of uptake of morphine into the circulation after injection into subcutaneous tissue is similar to the uptake following an IM injection, the dose, dose interval and guidelines for titration are the same as for IM morphine (see **Box 4.2**).

ORAL ADMINISTRATION

Delays in gastric emptying are common after surgery, injury and opioid administration. Because of this and the possibility of post-operative nausea and vomiting, the use of oral opioids for the treatment of moderate to severe acute pain has not been common practice. If gastric emptying is delayed the opioids will not pass through to the small intestine where they are absorbed. When emptying does occur, several doses may enter the small intestine at once. However, once a postoperative or post-injury patient is able to tolerate unrestricted amounts of oral fluids, gastric empty-ing is returning to normal and there is often no need to continue administration of parenteral opioids.

By the time a patient can take oral opioids after major surgery or injury, pain is often less intense and episodes of 'incident' pain less severe. Providing the differences between oral and parenteral doses are understood, oral opioids can be very effective. If a patient cannot swallow tablets, many of the opioids are available as an elixir.

Larger doses are required when opioids are given orally because of the 'first pass' effect. That is, the proportion of an orally administered drug that is metabolized by the liver and/or gut wall after absorption from the gastrointestinal tract determines the amount of unchanged drug that reaches the systemic circula-tion. The equianalgesic doses of oral and parenteral opioids are listed in **Box 2.5** in Chapter 2.

Slow or sustained release preparations of oral morphine are available for the treatment of chronic and cancer pain and only need to be given two or three times a day. The slower onset of action (2–3 hours to peak effect) makes them unsuitable for the treatment of acute pain. The long half-life of methadone makes it more difficult to titrate pain relief rapidly without risking accu-mulation of the drug, so it too is unsuitable for the routine management of acute pain.

TITRATION OF ORAL OPIOIDS

Titration of oral opioids is very similar to that of IM and SC opioids once allowances are made for equianalgesic doses.

Dose range

As for other routes of opioid administration, doses should be based on the age of the patient. If the patient has been receiving parenteral opioids, particularly via PCA, the parenteral opioid requirements can be used as a guide to the dose of oral opioid that is likely to be needed. If a dose – especially one based on prior parenteral opioid requirements – appears to have no effect, a continued delay in gastric emptying should be suspected and consideration given to returning to parenteral opioids.

Oxycodone and codeine are two opioids commonly given orally for the treatment of acute pain. The dose of oral oxycodone that is usually considered to be equianalgesic to 10 mg of parenteral morphine is 10–20 mg. However, possibly because acute pain, unlike chronic pain, decreases in severity each day, the equianalgesic dose is often clinically closer to 10 mg oral oxycodone (i.e. a ratio of 1:1). Oxycodone is often classed as a 'weak' opioid, but it is not. The amount that can be given orally is only limited by the number of tablets that a patient can reasonably be expected to swallow in one dose (usually no more than eight or ten, i.e. 40–50 mg). If formulations are used where oxycodone is combined with acetaminophen (paracetamol) or aspirin, it is the limits placed on the doses of these drugs that will limit the total amount of oxycodone that can be given in one day. It is recommended that doses of acetaminophen do not exceed 4 g per day. These recommendations may vary from one country to another.

Similarly, oral codeine is commonly administered in a tablet form that combines it with acetaminophen, and therefore the amount of opioid that can be given is limited.

Oral propoxyphene (dextropropoxyphene), again usually marketed in a combination formulation, is generally given only for the treatment of mild pain.

Dose interval

As with IM and SC regimens, oral opioids can be ordered PRN or at fixed-interval doses. The onset of action of oral opioids is a little slower than that of intermittent IM/SC injections and a PRN regimen may not be entirely successful, especially if pain is still moderate to severe and the dose required reasonably large. An alternative is to give the drug at a fixed interval (e.g. strictly 4-hourly), and vary the dose. This interval can be shorter than 4 hours if needed, or medication for breakthrough pain can be ordered in addition to the fixed-interval opioid. Knowledge of a patient's prior opioid requirements (e.g. if a patient is switching from PCA) makes fixed-interval dosing much easier, as it gives a good guide to the patient's likely 24-hour oral opioid requirement. Ideally, the patient should be allowed to choose the dose of opioid from the range ordered, based on the effect of previous doses.

Monitoring and selection of subsequent doses

Pain scores, sedation scores and respiratory rate should be monitored as for IM/SC opioids.

INTERMITTENT INTRAVENOUS ADMINISTRATION

Many books and guidelines still suggest that intravenous (IV) opioids should be given in doses similar to those administered intramuscularly and at similar dose intervals. **Figure 4.2** is a hypothetical representation of what might happen to opioid blood levels if the *same dose* of opioid administered by IM injection in **Figure 4.1** is given by IV injection every 4 hours. This regimen would result in large variations in the blood concentrations of the drug, and it is not a particularly effective way of administering opioids. If sustained pain relief is to be obtained without side effects, much smaller doses have to be given much more often. A protocol that has been widely used for the administration of intermittent IV bolus doses of opioid is reproduced in **Box 4.3**. It is managed by the nursing staff (usually in the post-anesthesia recovery areas or other specialized areas such as the burns unit),

- only to be used by staff who have been instructed in this technique •
- NOT appropriate for routine maintenance of analgesia in general wards •
- Note that the peak effect of an intravenous dose may not occur for over 15 minutes •
  so all patients should be observed closely during this time

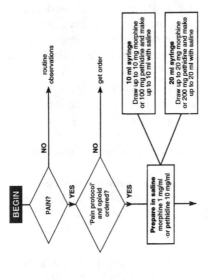

BEGIN

PAIN? —— NO —→ routine observations

YES
↓

'Pain protocol' and opioid ordered? —— NO —→ get order

YES
↓

Prepare in saline
morphine 1 mg/ml
or pethidine 10 mg/ml

10 ml syringe
Draw up to 10 mg morphine
or 100 mg pethidine and make
up to 10 ml with saline

20 ml syringe
Draw up to 20 mg morphine
or 200 mg pethidine and make
up to 20 ml with saline

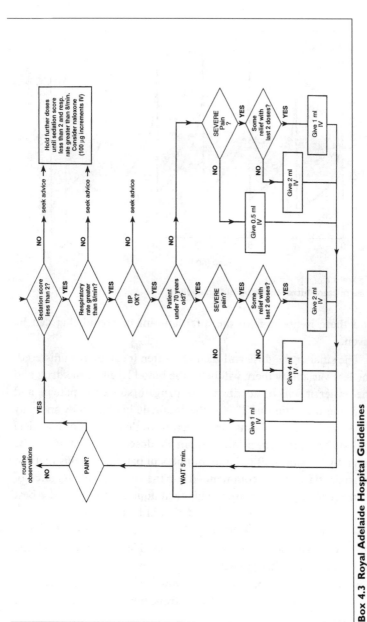

Box 4.3 Royal Adelaide Hospital Guidelines
INTERMITTENT INTRAVENOUS OPIOID ADMINISTRATION
for Acute Pain Management 1/1/95

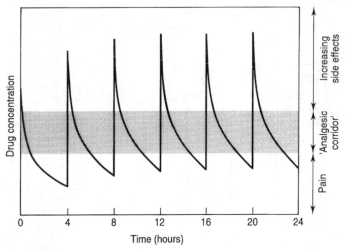

Figure 4.2
Intermittent intravenous opioid analgelsia

and there is no limit to the total amount of opioid that can be given.

The smaller the dose and the more often it can be administered, the less variability there will be in the blood levels of the drug and the easier it will be to titrate the drug to suit each patient and differing pain stimuli. This is the rationale behind PCA and why PCA has been so effective. However, it would be a major logistical and staffing problem if intermittent IV doses of opioid had to be given by nursing staff to large numbers of patients, so this method of analgesia is not recommended for the routine maintenance of pain relief in general wards. This technique is, however, the best way to obtain rapid analgesia and should be used to:

- obtain initial pain relief (e.g. immediately after an operation), i.e. 'load' the patient so that the blood levels rapidly reach the MEAC for that patient
- provide analgesia for patients who are hypovolemic or hypotensive, when uptake of drug from muscle or subcutaneous tissue is poor

---

▼ **Titration of intermittent intravenous opioids**

Requires:

An age-related range of morphine doses (suggested doses are examples only)	< 70 years: 1 mg, 2 mg or 4 mg > 70 years: 0.5 mg, 1 mg or 2 mg
An appropriate dose interval	3–5 minutes
Monitoring of pain score, sedation score and respiratory rate	see Box 4.3
Monitoring for presence of other side effects	
Selection of subsequent doses according to patient response	see Box 4.3

Aims for:
patient comfort, sedation score < 2 and respiratory rate > 8/minute

---

Box 4.4

- cover episodes of 'incident pain' (e.g. dressing changes, physiotherapy) or inadequate analgesia

TITRATION OF INTERMITTENT IV OPIOIDS

Dose range

As before, dose ranges should be based on the age of the patient. Doses outlined in **Box 4.4** are reduced for patients over 70 years old.

Dose interval

It may take 15 minutes or more for a less lipid-soluble drug like morphine to exert its maximum effect on the central nervous system after IV administration. However, this interval is too long if analgesia is to be obtained rapidly. A reasonable balance between absolute safety (ensuring one dose has had its peak effect before another dose is given) and efficacy is to use a dose interval of 3–5 minutes. This has proved safe and very effective, as long as staff monitor the patient carefully and are aware that this interval may not represent the true time to peak effect.

Monitoring and selection of subsequent doses

A protocol is given in **Box 4.3**. While the protocol in **Box 4.3** is in use and for 15 minutes after cessation of the protocol, a nurse remains with the patient.

Subsequent analgesic regimens

Patients given intermittent IV opioids will normally be changed to an alternative analgesic regimen once comfortable. If PCA is to be used it can be started immediately. If IM or SC opioids are ordered a dose should be given at the earliest sign of discomfort.

CONTINUOUS INTRAVENOUS INFUSIONS

In an attempt to avoid the 'peaks and troughs' in blood concentration associated with intermittent administration, continuous intravenous infusions of opioid are sometimes used for the management of acute pain. While it may be possible to maintain reasonably constant blood levels using this technique, it is difficult to predict what the level will need to be for a particular patient or what dose is needed to achieve it. Also, acute pain is not constant and the amount of opioid required by a patient will vary in response to different pain stimuli. For the reasons outlined below, alterations of infusion rate alone will often mean there is a considerable delay in matching the amount of opioid delivered to the amount of opioid actually needed. There are also possible risks from blood levels of the drug that may continue to rise after analgesia has been obtained.

If an infusion of any drug is ordered at a fixed rate, it takes five half-lives of the drug to reach 95% of the final steady state concentration. The half-life of morphine is 2–3 hours, so it may take up to 15 hours for blood levels to plateau at this steady state concentration. It is this plateau that needs to be in the 'analgesic corridor'.

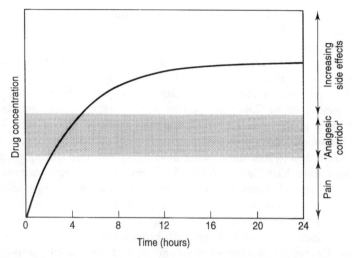

Figure 4.3
Continuous intravenous opioid infusions

It can been seen from the hypothetical representation in **Figure 4.3** of a continuous infusion of an opioid with a half-life of 3 hours (e.g. morphine or meperidine), that analgesia is obtained within 3 hours of starting the infusion. If this infusion continues at the same rate, the blood concentration will continue to rise for some hours, and side effects (including respiratory depression) may result. It will also take some hours for each alteration made to the infusion rate to have its full effect, i.e. to reach the new steady state concentration – a fact often not recognized by staff who change the rates as often as every 30 minutes.

If patients become sedated while using PCA (PCA mode only) they will not press the demand button and further doses of opioid will not be delivered. Equipment used for continuous infusions of opioid will continue to deliver the drug regardless of whether the patient is sedated or not. For this reason continuous intravenous opioid infusions are probably the *least safe* way to administer opioids in a general ward. They should only be used where close observation of the patient can be guaranteed.

TITRATION OF CONTINUOUS IV OPIOID INFUSIONS

Dose range

In view of the variable time taken from the commencement of a continuous infusion to the onset of pain relief, analgesia will be obtained more rapidly if IV bolus doses (as in **Box 4.4**) are administered to 'load' the patient in the first instance and the infusion is commenced only when the patient is comfortable. It has been said that the rate of the infusion can then be based on this loading dose – half the loading dose being required during each elimination half-life. However, half-lives vary between patients; various opioid doses may have been given during the operative period; pain immediately after surgery may be different from pain later in the ward (e.g. shoulder tip pain after laparoscopy or abdominal colic may have abated); sedation after anesthesia may have limited the amount of opioid given; and the volume status of the patient may have altered (hypovolemia reducing the amount of opioid needed). These and other variables make this calculation, at best, a guide only.

Monitoring

Sedation scores, pain scores and respiratory rates should be monitored frequently, and hourly intervals are suggested.

Alterations of infusion rates

Because of the time taken for any alterations in infusion rate to have an effect, if analgesia is inadequate, IV bolus doses should again be used to achieve patient comfort before the infusion rate is increased.

If an infusion is stopped it will also take five half-lives of the drug to return to a blood concentration of zero. Therefore, if a patient becomes oversedated, the infusion should cease until the patient is more awake (sedation score less than 2), not merely reduced to a lower rate.

CONTINUOUS SUBCUTANEOUS INFUSIONS

Continuous subcutaneous infusions of opioid are commonly used in the management of cancer pain but they have also been used in the treatment of acute pain. Absorption from the subcutaneous site means that the onset of analgesia and the time taken to see the effects from any changes in infusion rates will be slower than for IV infusions, but the two techniques are otherwise very similar.

RECTAL ADMINISTRATION

The submucosal venous plexus of the rectum drains into the superior, middle and inferior rectal veins. Drug absorbed from the lower half of the rectum will pass into the latter two veins and into the inferior vena cava, thus bypassing the portal vein and 'first pass' metabolism in the liver. This is one of the advantages of this route of administration. Drug absorbed through the rectal mucosa of the upper part of the rectum passes into the superior rectal vein and does enter the portal system.

Rectal absorption is often very variable owing to differences in the site of placement of the drug, the contents of the rectum and the blood supply to the rectum. In addition, there is not always widespread patient – or indeed staff – acceptance of this route of administration. The drug may not be distributed evenly through-out the suppository and therefore doses of 'half a suppository' may not deliver half of the amount of opioid in that suppository.

REFERENCES AND FURTHER READING

Austin K.L., Stapleton J.V. and Mather L.E. (1980) Multiple intramuscular injections: a major source of variability in analgesic response to meperidine. *Pain* **8**, 47–62.

Hanning C.D. (1990) The rectal absorption of opioids. In *Advances in Pain Research and Therapy* (Volume 14): *Opioid Analgesia* (eds Benedetti C., Chapman C.R. and Giron G.). Raven Press, New York.

Lasagna L. and Beecher H.K. (1954) The optimal dose of morphine. *Journal of the American Medical Association* **156**, 230–234.

Levy M.H. (1990) Oral controlled release morphine: guidelines for clinical use. In *Advances in Pain Research and Therapy* (Volume 14): *Opioid Analgesia* (eds Benedetti C., Chapman C.R. and Giron G.). Raven Press, New York.

Thirlwell M.P., Boos G.J. and Hollingsworth M.L. (1990) Clinical pharmacokinetics of oral controlled release morphine: an overview. In *Advances in Pain Research and Therapy* (Volume 14): *Opioid Analgesia* (eds Benedetti C., Chapman C.R. and Giron G.). Raven Press, New York.

CHAPTER 5

PATIENT-CONTROLLED ANALGESIA

The concept of patient-controlled analgesia (PCA);

Contraindications;

PCA variables;

Monitoring;

Standard orders and nursing policies and protocols;

Daily management;

Subsequent analgesic regimens;

Complications;

Alternative routes;

The opioid-tolerant patient

THE CONCEPT OF PATIENT-CONTROLLED ANALGESIA (PCA)

Patient-controlled analgesia, in a broad sense, is not restricted to a single route or method of analgesic administration or a single class of analgesic drug, but means that patients can determine when and how much analgesic they receive. However, the term PCA is more commonly used to describe a method of analgesia which employs sophisticated infusion devices and allows patients to self-administer opioids, usually intravenously.

In 1968 Sechzer noted, in a publication concerning the measurement of pain, that good postoperative analgesia could be obtained using repeated small bolus doses of an intravenous opioid administered by a nurse-observer following a patient demand (Sechzer, 1968). He and others subsequently developed machines that enabled the patient to self-administer small intravenous bolus doses of opioid when required. In the early 1970s the first commercially available PCA machines were released, but PCA continued to be used primarily as a research tool. Although more effective than conventional intermittent opioid regimens in a general ward setting, PCA has only come into widespread and worldwide use in the last few years, following a more organized approach to acute pain management and the introduction of acute pain services.

Compared with conventional intermittent opioid regimens, any regimen that uses small and frequent intravenous bolus doses of opioid given as often as needed, such as PCA, is more likely to maintain a reasonably constant blood concentration of the drug, a concentration that could be kept within the 'analgesic corridor' for each patient (**Figure 5.1**).

In addition, PCA has other advantages:

- the flexibility of PCA helps to overcome the wide interpatient variation in opioid requirements (eightfold to tenfold) in each age group (see chapter 2)

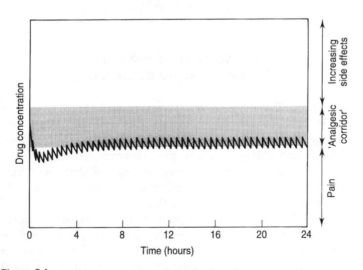

Figure 5.1
Patient-controlled analgesia is more likely to maintain blood concentrations of the drug within the 'analgesic corridor'

- patients can receive additional opioid whenever they become uncomfortable. With conventional nurse-administered opioid regimens patients will often not request another dose until pain is severe. They must then endure the inevitable delays before the dose is given and the time for the drug to take effect
- the intensity of acute pain is rarely constant, and PCA means that the amount of opioid delivered can be rapidly titrated according to increases and decreases in the pain stimulus within each patient
- while side effects may occur as a result of opioid administration, PCA enables patients to titrate the amount of opioid delivered against both pain and dose-related side effects

Most PCA systems incorporate microprocessor-driven syringe pumps that, within preset limits, will deliver a bolus dose of a drug when the patient presses a demand button connected to the pump. Access to the syringe (or other drug reservoir) and the microprocessor program are only possible using a key or an access code. Certain variables are prescribed and programmed into the PCA machine which control how much opioid the patient can receive. Most machines can also deliver a continuous or 'background' infusion, thus PCA machines can operate in three modes:

- PCA mode only
- continuous infusion only
- a combination of PCA with a continuous (background) infusion

Patients using PCA are instructed to push the demand button whenever they are uncomfortable. Where the patient is unable to use either hand, if the PCA machine has a pneumatic demand mechanism a piece of plastic tubing can be attached to the machine instead of the hand-held button and the patient instructed to blow into this tubing. Some machines will also operate with a pressure-sensitive pad or foot pedal.

More recently, small disposable PCA devices have been developed. These deliver a fixed volume so that the concentration of drug in the reservoir must be changed if increases or decreases in the size of the incremental bolus dose are required. Unlike other PCA machines, the drug reservoir is easily accessible.

The inherent safety of the technique lies in the fact that, as long as the machine is in PCA mode only (i.e. there is no continuous infusion), no further doses of opioid will be delivered should the patient become sedated, because no further demands will be made. This assumes that the patient is the only one pressing the button. Staff must explain to the patient, relatives and friends that no-one but the patient is allowed to operate the PCA machine.

Many institutions will have only a few PCA machines. Patients who will benefit from PCA most are those who have had major surgery and are not permitted oral fluids (and who therefore cannot take oral analgesics), those with marked 'incident' pain (e.g. associated with physiotherapy or dressing changes) and those who cannot be given intramuscular injections even for a short time (e.g. hemophiliac patients). The PCA machines are most commonly used for intravenous opioid administration but can also be used to deliver analgesics via subcutaneous or epidural routes.

CONTRAINDICATIONS

A current or past history of addiction to opioid drugs was often thought to be a contraindication to PCA. It is now realized that PCA can be a very useful way of managing acute pain in this population, when supervised by pain specialists. Much larger opioid doses than usual will often be required.

Recognized contraindications to the use of PCA are discussed below (**Box 5.1**).

UNTRAINED NURSING AND MEDICAL STAFF
Patient-controlled analgesia should not be used by medical or nursing staff who have not had the appropriate training. Using PCA is a very effective way of providing good analgesia, but the results depend on a good understanding of the technique. An inadequate understanding of PCA, the drugs and doses used, the monitoring requirements and the management of common problems can, at worst, increase the risk of complications. At

Contraindications to PCA
Untrained staff (nursing and medical) Patient rejection Patient inability to comprehend the technique (e.g. language barrier, confusion) ? Extremes of age

Box 5.1

best, it can prove to be a very expensive way of providing poor analgesia. In many institutions the use of PCA is supervised by anesthesiologists.

Nursing education and accreditation programs that have to be completed by each nurse before he or she can take responsibility for a patient with PCA are recommended. If this is done, there is no reason why nursing staff cannot take responsibility for programming the PCA machines, changing the syringes or making alterations to the program according to guidelines in the PCA orders.

PATIENT REJECTION

The majority of patients appreciate the control that PCA gives them and the ability to rapidly titrate their own analgesia and balance pain relief with the degree of any side effects that may occur. This is one of the reasons why patients using PCA sometimes express a greater satisfaction with this technique compared with others such as epidural analgesia, even though the degree of pain relief may be less. Some patients, however, do not want this control and prefer the nursing and medical staff to manage the analgesia. With these patients, PCA therapy will often fail.

INABILITY TO COMPREHEND THE TECHNIQUE

For PCA to be used both safely and effectively the patient must be able to understand the technique. Patients should not automatically be excluded from consideration if there is mild mental impairment or a language barrier. Relatives or translators can be asked to interpret verbal instructions about the use of PCA and patient education leaflets can be written in any language. However, if staff feel that despite these measures the patient still does not understand PCA, alternative methods of pain relief will be needed. Patients who are confused should not be offered PCA and those who become confused should have PCA discontinued.

An understanding of PCA does not necessarily have to be detailed as long as it is safe. Some elderly patients have thought that the hand-held button contained a 'magic beam' and needed to be directed at the site of the pain before being pressed (problems only arise if they attempt to treat other patients' pain as well!); some have used the button as they would a bronchodilator inhaler, that is, when they require another dose they bring the button to their mouth, press it and inhale! As long as they are aware that the button is pressed only when they become uncomfortable, the patient should be allowed to continue with PCA.

PATIENT AGE
The technique has been used successfully in patients of all ages. Children as young as 4 years old and patients in their 90s can manage PCA very well as long as they understand the explanations given and are willing to be active participants in their own care.

PCA VARIABLES

There are many different models of PCA machine now available. Although the variables that can be programmed into the machines differ a little, there are a number of features that are common to most or all of them.

LOADING DOSE
Patient-controlled analgesia is a maintenance therapy and will not be effective if moderate or severe pain is present when it commences, as the patient is unlikely to be able to obtain enough opioid within a short period to achieve an adequate degree of comfort. To make the patient comfortable before PCA is started, a loading dose of the opioid is needed. There is an enormous interpatient variation in the amount of opioid required

as a loading dose and it may be better to individualize this dose for each patient (e.g. by using the protocol in **Box 4.3** in Chapter 4), rather than program a single loading dose via the PCA machine.

INCREMENTAL (BOLUS) DOSE

The bolus dose is the amount of opioid (in milligrams or micrograms) that the PCA machine will deliver when the demand button is pressed. Many opioids have been used with PCA (morphine being the most common) but those with very short or very long durations of action are not recommended. Partial agonist or agonist-antagonist opioids are used far less commonly than pure opioid agonists.

The size of the incremental dose, along with the lock-out interval (see below), can determine the effectiveness of PCA. If the dose is too small many patients will be unable to obtain adequate analgesia; if the dose is too large there may be an unacceptable incidence of side effects. Commonly used initial dose sizes are given in Box 5.2. The optimal incremental dose for each patient would be one that consistently results in appreciable analgesia without side effects. Therefore, adjustments to the size of the initial dose prescribed may be required.

With conventional intermittent opioid regimens, the dose of opioid prescribed should be reduced as the age of the patient increases. As patients with PCA can vary the total daily dose according to the number of demands they make, a progressive decrease in dose with increasing age is not necessary. However, patients over 70 years old will have, on average, less than half the total daily opioid requirements of a 20-year-old, and it is reasonable to start with smaller (e.g. half) PCA incremental doses.

DOSE DURATION

The rate at which the PCA machine delivers the bolus dose can be altered in some machines allowing the bolus dose to be delivered as an infusion (e.g. over 5 minutes). If subcutaneous PCA is used (see later), rapid delivery of a dose may cause some stinging and a slower rate of delivery will reduce the chance of this occurring.

LOCK-OUT INTERVAL

The time from the *end* of the delivery of one dose until the machine will respond to another demand is called the 'lock-out' interval. This is to allow the effect of one dose to be felt before another can be given and is one of the safety features of the machine. Lock-out intervals of 5–8 minutes are commonly prescribed, regardless of the drug used. Even though it may theoretically take up to 15 minutes or longer for the peak effect of an intravenous dose of morphine to be seen, in practice it is difficult to discern any major differences between the onset times of the commonly used opioids. A longer lock-out, waiting for the maximum effect of the drug in all cases, would reduce the ability of the patient to rapidly titrate the amount of opioid required and would therefore decrease the effectiveness of PCA.

When patients are told about the lock-out interval, it is important to make sure that they realize it only means the time interval that elapses before another dose *can* be delivered, should they press the button, and *not* that they need to press every 5 or 8 minutes!

Lock-out intervals of 5–8 minutes mean that, allowing for the time for the dose to be delivered, a patient could demand and receive up to ten doses of the opioid each hour. In reality, if patients feel that a particular incremental dose is not effective they will not continue to press the demand button. Most patients have an inherent maximum frequency of demand, and it is uncommon for a patient to sustain a demand rate of more than three or four doses each hour. If, despite an average of three or four doses per hour, analgesia is inadequate, the bolus dose should be increased rather than the 'lock-out' interval decreased or the patient instructed to press the button more often.

CONTINUOUS (BACKGROUND) INFUSION

In most PCA machines a continuous infusion can be delivered with or without the patient demand mode. It was hoped that by using a continuous infusion of opioid at a low rate, a constant but sub-analgesic blood concentration could be maintained. Therefore, when a bolus dose of opioid was delivered, the blood level would reach the 'analgesic corridor' more rapidly. It was also hoped that the continuous infusion would enable the patient to make fewer demands, sleep for longer periods and wake in less pain.

Unfortunately, there is no consistent evidence to suggest that the routine addition of a continuous infusion to PCA has had the beneficial effects that were anticipated for the average opioid naive patient. It does not always reduce the number of demands made by the patient but does increase the total amount of opioid delivered; it has been shown to increase the risk of side effects, including respiratory depression; and it does not always result in better analgesia or improved sleep patterns. A continuous infusion reduces the inherent safety of the PCA technique as it will be delivered regardless of the sedation level of the patient. In addition, the incidence of pump programming errors is greater when the continuous infusion mode is used, adding to the risk of excessive doses being delivered. The routine use of a continuous infusion with PCA, especially before a patient's opioid requirements are known, is therefore not recommended.

However, there may be benefits to be gained from the use of a continuous infusion in addition to PCA mode in patients who are tolerant to opioids (for definitions see Chapter 1) or in those who complain of waking in severe pain at night. In both these situations the opioid requirement of the patient is likely to be known and the rate of infusion can be adjusted accordingly. Patients needing PCA for long periods (e.g. burns patients or those with oral mucositis following bone marrow transplantation) may benefit from continuous infusion at night. Once again, the opioid requirements of each patient will be known and the infusion rate can be calculated according to those requirements. A typical approach is to order a continuous infusion that provides 30–50% of a patient's *known* hourly opioid dose.

Usually, if the combination of a continuous infusion and PCA mode is prescribed in opioid-naive patients, it is recommended that the rate in milligrams per hour should be no more than the size of the bolus dose in milligrams.

CONCENTRATION

For consistency and safety, each institution should standardize the concentrations of drugs administered by PCA. Where possible, syringes and other drug reservoirs should be prefilled in the pharmacy. Most companies that manufacture PCA machines suggest that the volume delivered following each demand should not be less than 0.5 ml.

HOURLY OR 4-HOURLY LIMITS

The hourly or 4-hourly limit, not present on all machines, is designed as a safety feature and prevents the patient receiving more than a designated amount of opioid within this time. However, very large interpatient variations in opioid requirements make it impossible to predict the 'safe' limit for each patient.

A commonly prescribed limit is 30 mg of morphine (or equianalgesic doses of an alternative opioid) in 4 hours. This may be

▼

Commonly prescribed initial values for PCA variables

Variable	Value	Comments
● Loading dose	0 mg (i.e. zero)	Best to titrate for each patient *before* starting PCA
● Incremental dose (bolus dose)	Morphine 1 mg Meperidine 10 mg Diamorphine 0.5–1 mg Fentanyl 20 µg Hydromorphone 0.2 mg	Consider starting with doses half these amounts in patients over 70 years old
● Concentration	Variable	Best if standardized for each drug
● Dose duration	Cannot be adjusted in most PCA machines, but where this can be done 'stat' is the shortest dose duration	
● Lock-out period	5–8 minutes	
● Background infusion	0 mg/hr (i.e. zero)	See text for exceptions
● 1-hour or 4-hour limits	30 mg morphine (or equivalent) in 4 hours	Consider varying according to patient age

Box 5.2

inadequate for some patients yet may be all that others require in 24 hours. For PCA to be used effectively, a wide range of opioid requirements need to be recognized and tolerated. The setting of a dose limit may not mean added safety for those patients with low opioid requirements, and may prevent those needing higher doses from obtaining good pain relief. The exception to this is meperidine, where doses should be limited to levels not associated with normeperidine toxicity.

The setting of a limit may give staff a false sense of security, as they may believe that the patient cannot receive an excessive dose of drug. As with other features designed to increase patient safety with PCA, the setting of a dose limit cannot compensate for any shortcomings in monitoring by ward staff.

Commonly used settings for PCA variables are listed in **Box 5.2**.

MONITORING

As in any opioid regimen used for the management of acute pain, pain score, sedation score and respiratory rate should be monitored. These should be recorded at regular intervals, along with the total amount of opioid delivered, the dose of any drug administered for the treatment of side effects, and any changes that have been made to the PCA program. Pain scores can be omitted if the patient is asleep, but an assessment of sedation must still be made. A sleeping patient who stirs when spoken to or touched is 'rousable' (with a sedation score of 'S'), and it is not necessary to wake the patient fully. Monitoring requirements need not increase the workload of the ward nursing staff. For example, while observations every 1–2 hours are recommended for the first 8 hours after PCA is commenced, this interval can be increased to 2–4 hourly thereafter, if the patient is stable.

The monitoring and recording of these parameters allows for a regular assessment of the progress of each patient and for rational changes to be made to the PCA orders so that treatment is individualized. It should be noted that most patients will titrate their pain relief to a level at which they are comfortable and not aim for complete analgesia, even in the absence of opioid-related side effects. Examples of flowsheets used for the recording of this information are included in the appendix at the end of this chapter.

Certain higher-risk patients, such as the morbidly obese and those with sleep apnea or severe obstructive pulmonary disease, will require additional and closer observation during the first 24 hours using PCA. Continuous pulse oximetry should be considered.

STANDARD ORDERS AND NURSING POLICIES AND PROTOCOLS

To maximize the effectiveness of PCA and minimize the risk of complications, standard orders and nursing policies and protocols are recommended.

STANDARD ORDERS
Standard orders need to cover a number of different areas, as follows.

Nondrug treatment orders
Nondrug treatment orders may include a statement to eliminate the concurrent ordering of CNS depressants or other opioids by others; orders for oxygen; the need for a one-way 'antireflux' valve to be sited in the IV line (to prevent the opioid travelling back up the primary IV line should the IV cannula become obstructed); availability of drugs to treat side effects; monitoring and documentation requirements; and information about the person to contact if problems occur.

PCA orders
All variables of the PCA program need to be prescribed. Additionally, it is helpful to have orders that enable staff to increase or decrease the size of the bolus dose if needed.

Orders for the treatment of side effects
There will always be some patients who suffer from one or more of

the side effects of opioids. The inclusion of standard orders for the recognition and management of these side effects will minimize delays in treatment.

To standardize the orders throughout the institution, preprinted forms are recommended. The important elements that should be included in these forms are listed in **Box 5.3**. The forms need to be completed and then signed and dated by the treating doctor.

Examples of preprinted pain management flow sheets and PCA standard orders are included in the appendix at the end of this chapter.

Important elements of intravenous PCA preprinted orders

1. *Drug(s), concentration(s)*
2. *Pump settings* — Incremental dose
   Lock-out interval
   Other limits (e.g. 4 hour, 1 hour)
3. *Mode of use* — PCA only
   Continuous infusion
4. *Initial drug loading instructions*
5. *Instructions for treating breakthrough pain*
6. *A statement to eliminate the ordering of CNS depressants by others*
7. *Monitoring instructions*
8. *Availability of drugs to treat side effects*
9. *Instructions for the treatment of side effects* — Respiratory depression
   Nausea and/or vomiting
   Pruritus
   Urinary retention
10. *Instructions about concurrent use of other CNS depressants*
11. *Instructions about whom to contact if problems occur*
12. *Date, time, signature*

Reproduced from Ready et al (1995) with permission

Box 5.3

▼ Elements of intravenous PCA nursing policies and protocols

1. A statement of the institution policy towards accreditation for nursing staff responsible for a patient with PCA.
2. A statement indicating who has responsibility for writing PCA orders.
3. The location of keys for PCA machines (usually with Controlled Substances keys).
4. Mechanisr.ıs for the checking and discarding of PCA opioids.
5. Guidelines for the suitability, or otherwise, of patients for PCA.
6. Instructions and guidelines for preoperative patient education.
7. Monitoring and documentation requirements.
8. Availability and use of drugs to treat side effects.
9. Instructions for the checking of the PCA settings against the prescription (e.g. at each shift change and change of syringe).
10. Instructions for checking the amount of drug delivered (from the machine display) against the amount remaining in the syringe.
11. Detailed instruction on the setting up and programming of the PCA machine.
12. The use of a one-way antireflux valve.
13. Management of equipment faults and alarms.
14. Instructions about whom to call if assistance or advice is required.

Box 5.4

NURSING PROCEDURE PROTOCOLS

The format of nursing procedure protocols for PCA will vary with each institution, but there are elements that need to be included in each, regardless of format. These are listed in **Box 5.4**.

DAILY MANAGEMENT

Standard orders are used for the initial prescription of PCA but these orders may not be effective for all patients. Daily evaluation (or more often if required) will allow assessment of the effectiveness of PCA and the treatment of side effects, including the need for changes to the PCA prescription or additional/alternative

Elements of intravenous PCA daily care

The following items should be included during a bedside evaluation at least once a day while intravenous PCA is administered.

1. **Note** the dose of analgesic medication given in the past 24 hours, and parameters of PCA settings (PCA bolus dose, lock-out interval, basal infusion if applicable, hourly or other interval limit).

2. **Evaluate** pain intensity both at rest and with operation-specific convalescent activity (e.g. passive continuous movement for knee replacement or chest physical therapy for thoracotomy). If pain is out of proportion to the surgical procedure, the number of days elapsed postoperatively and analgesic therapy given, consider whether another cause is present (e.g. surgical complication, personality disorder, opioid tolerance) and initiate appropriate evaluation, including communication with the surgeon and/or other consultant physicians.

3. **Determine** whether side effects are present. Assess each side effect, e.g. sedation, in the context of the type of operation and days elapsed since the operation. Decide whether the side effect is in proportion to the operation, the number of days postoperatively, and the amount of opioid and other medications given. For sedation, as an example, note other concurrent drug therapy and decide whether to undertake additional tests (e.g. assessment of glucose, electrolytes, arterial blood gas, calcium, magnesium, electrocardiogram).

4. **Perform** a problem-oriented physical examination (e.g. surgical site, presence of rales, venous thrombosis). Note the current vital signs (heart rate, respiratory rate, blood pressure) and compare them with the last evaluation. If these are unstable or unsatisfactory (e.g. low blood pressure or irregular pulse), consider suitable diagnostic investigations (e.g. hematocrit, electrocardiogram).

5. **Consider** whether the patient would benefit from changing the PCA pump settings or the PCA opioid.

6. **Note** concurrent medications and consider whether the patient would benefit from changing the overall regimen (e.g. simplifying to avert drug interactions), or employing adjuvant analgesic medication or nonpharmacological therapies, and if so, order these.

7. **Evaluate** overall patient satisfaction with current care.

8. **Evaluate** patient's responses to prior adjustments of pain therapy or addition of adjuvants (e.g. for nausea or anxiety).

---

9. **Evaluate** patient's suitability for making the transition to simpler alternatives (e.g. oral analgesics).
10. **Discuss** the assessment and plan with the patient and the patient's nurse and/or surgeon when appropriate.
11. **Document** findings, impression and plan in the hospital chart.
12. **Ensure** availability of personnel with appropriate expertise to deal with questions or problems at any time.

Box 5.5
Reproduced from Ready et al (1995) with permission

analgesic techniques; an overall assessment of the patient, including the possibility of non-PCA-related complications and any concurrent medication orders; and discussion with the patient and the patient's nurse and/or doctor of the assessment and treatment plans.

Advantage should be taken of the opportunity to encourage patients and staff to use the pain relief provided by PCA to exercise and mobilize – better analgesia alone will not necessarily improve patient outcome.

Guidelines for daily evaluation of PCA suggested by the American Society of Anesthesiologists are listed in **Box 5.5**.

SUBSEQUENT ANALGESIC REGIMENS

Opioid requirements during PCA can be used as guide for the opioid regimen once PCA has ceased. If the patient is allowed (and tolerating) unlimited oral fluids, oral opioids can be ordered. If PCA must cease before oral fluids can be given, other parenteral (intramuscular, subcutaneous or intravenous) opioids will be needed. In general, PCA should be maintained until oral opioids can be used.

There should be some overlap of pain therapies so that the subsequent regimen has time to have an effect before PCA is stopped. If there is to be a change in clinician responsibility for the pain management of the patient, then this change needs to be clearly understood by all staff.

ORAL OPIOIDS

Any of the oral opioids suitable for the management of acute pain may be used following PCA (see Chapter 4). The dose of oral opioid to be prescribed is based on the amount of opioid used in the 24 hours prior to stopping PCA and the equianalgesic doses of the PCA and oral opioids (Chapter 2). For example, if oral oxycodone is prescribed to follow IV morphine PCA, the daily oxycodone requirements will be about the same as the previous 24-hour morphine requirements. To allow patients the ability to titrate their own analgesia, it is best to allow the daily oxycodone dose to range between half and twice the last 24-hour PCA morphine requirement. The estimated 24-hour oxycodone dose can then be ordered in six divided doses. As an example:

> if immediate last 24-hour PCA morphine = 60 mg
> then next 24-hour oxycodone requirements = 30 mg to 120 mg
> therefore order = 5 mg to 20 mg 4-hourly

If PCA morphine requirements are less than about 30 mg per day, less potent formulations such as a combination of acetaminophen (paracetamol) and codeine may suffice. Other analgesics, such as nonsteroidal anti-inflammatory drugs (NSAIDs) may also be used.

INTRAMUSCULAR (IM) OR SUBCUTANEOUS (SC) OPIOIDS

To convert PCA morphine requirements to an intermittent IM or SC regimen, the 24-hour PCA dose can be divided by 8 to give the center of an appropriate dose range. As an example:

> immediate last 24-hour PCA morphine = 60 mg
> therefore, middle of dose range for IM/SC = 60 mg ÷ 8
> = 7.5 mg
> therefore order = 5 mg to 10 mg 2-hourly PRN

Although division by 8 assumes a 3-hourly dose, it is reasonable to add flexibility by ordering the range of doses 2-hourly PRN (see Chapter 4).

COMPLICATIONS

Complications of PCA may be related to the equipment, inadequate analgesia or the side effects of the opioids.

PROBLEMS RELATED TO THE EQUIPMENT

Equipment malfunction

Interference from current surges or static electricity has led to the deprogramming of some PCA machines. Usually this will be 'failsafe' – for example, the program will default to the lowest setting possible for a bolus dose. However, cases have been recorded where deprogramming of the PCA machine led to the continuous delivery of the contents of the syringe. To minimize the risk of deprogramming in machines subject to these problems, it is wise to check the PCA program whenever the syringe is changed and whenever the machine is connected to or disconnected from mains power (most machines have a battery 'back-up' that will enable the machine to run for up to 8 hours in the event of a power failure).

Cracked syringe barrels have enabled the contents of the PCA syringe to empty by gravity.

Operator error

Operator error can lead to misprogramming of the PCA machine, improper loading of the syringe or incorrect placement of the one-way antireflux valve. Failure to clamp the IV tubing during a syringe change may allow delivery of an inadvertent bolus dose of opioid. Errors in PCA prescriptions have also occurred – either inadvertently or due to an inadequate knowledge of PCA.

Non-patient activation of PCA

Respiratory depression has been reported following activation of PCA by well-meaning relatives or friends of the patient. Administration of doses by hospital staff, including nurses and physiotherapists, has also been reported. Except in special circumstances, this practice should be discouraged.

native ordered. If a patient has low opioid requirements, a decrease in the size of the bolus dose can also be tried. Patients who complain of a wave of nausea and dizziness a few minutes after pressing the demand button may benefit from a smaller bolus dose or a slower rate of infusion of the bolus dose (i.e. an increase in the 'dose duration').

Although there is little evidence to support a difference in the incidence of nausea and vomiting with different opioids, individual patients may appear to be more sensitive to one particular drug. In this case and if other measures have failed, a change to another opioid is worth considering. It may also be that the opioid is not the cause, or the sole cause, of the nausea and vomiting (see Chapter 2).

As the emetic effects of opioids are enhanced by vestibular

Sedation and respiratory depression
Sedation score 2, respiratory rate > 8/min: reduce (e.g. halve) size of bolus
  dose
Sedation score 2, respiratory rate < 8/min: reduce size of bolus dose,
  consider naloxone (100 μg)
Sedation score 3 (regardless of respiratory rate): administer naloxone
  (100 μg, repeat PRN)

Urinary retention
Catheterize – 'in-out' or indwelling

Confusion
May not be related to the opioid but PCA should cease and alternative
  analgesia given

Normeperidine toxicity (norpethidine)
Prevention is preferred by limiting total dose of meperidine administered

Decreased bowel motility
Anticipatory treatment where possible, and discourage use of PCA to cover
  discomfort resulting from resumption of peristalsis

Hypotension
Look for causes of hypovolemia

Box 5.6 (continued)

stimulation, the patient may feel better lying flat and minimizing movement until the treatment has taken effect. Transdermal scopolamine is often beneficial in this situation but is best avoided in patients over 60 years old.

Pruritus

As outlined in Chapter 2, pruritus may be due to histamine release or be a consequence of possible μ receptor activation. It is more common following administration of morphine than meperidine (pethidine) or fentanyl.

If a patient is disturbed by this side effect, the safest treatment in the first instance is to change to another opioid. Antihistamines, because of their sedative effects, may add to the risk of sedation and respiratory depression. The pruritus may also respond to small, carefully titrated doses of intravenous naloxone, but there is a risk that the naloxone may also reverse some of the analgesic effect of the opioid. Nalbuphine in small IV doses is sometimes effective.

Sedation and respiratory depression

The best clinical indicator of early respiratory depression is sedation. If a patient has a sedation score of 2 (frequently or constantly drowsy but is still easy to rouse, e.g. the patient wakes easily but is unable to stay awake during a conversation) but a respiratory rate above 8 per minute, a reduction in the size of the PCA bolus dose (e.g. by 50%) is usually indicated. Even if sedatives have been given this may still be the safest course of action – the dose can always be increased again if analgesia is inadequate once the patient is less sedated.

If the patient has a sedation score of 2 and a respiratory rate below 8 per minute, the administration of a small dose of naloxone (100 μg IV) should be considered in addition to a reduction in the size of the bolus dose. Whether or not naloxone is considered necessary in this instance may depend on factors such as staffing levels. If no nurse is available to keep a continued close watch on the patient, it may be safer to give naloxone. If a patient develops severe respiratory depression with a sedation score of 3 (unrousable), naloxone should be given regardless of the respiratory rate. Remember that naloxone has a shorter half-life than the commonly used opioid agonists, and repeated doses may be needed.

Respiratory depression during PCA therapy has been reported in patients following postoperative hemorrhage. A normally appropriate incremental dose of an opioid may become excessive in the presence of hypovolemia. Until the patient is normovolemic, smaller incremental bolus doses may be needed.

Urinary retention

Urinary retention may occur as a result of opioid administration. Whatever the cause, the patient may need to be catheterized – either an 'in-out' or indwelling catheter.

Confusion

Opioids will not usually be the cause, or the sole cause, of confusion. However, PCA needs to be discontinued as the patient may press the demand button inappropriately. Alternative methods of pain relief should be organized.

Normeperidine (norpethidine) toxicity

As described in Chapter 2, normeperidine toxicity can follow the administration of large doses of meperidine. This is more likely following PCA than conventional opioid techniques, as PCA has allowed some patients to receive more opioid than they would have done with nurse-administered analgesic regimens in the past. To minimize the risk of toxicity it is recommended that the total dose of meperidine delivered be kept to less than 1000 mg in the first 24 hours of therapy and less than 600–700 mg per day thereafter in the younger patient, and even less in the older patient or those with renal impairment.

Inhibition of bowel motility

To a greater or lesser extent inhibition of bowel motility is an inevitable consequence of the use of opioids. Where possible, and if opioids are to be used for some days, treatment should be anticipatory. Occasionally, patients may use PCA opioids to cover the often vague abdominal discomfort ('windy pains' or 'gas cramps') related to the resumption of peristalsis, e.g. after abdominal surgery, but the use of opioids in this way will further inhibit the return of bowel function. The patient should be encouraged to mobilize rather than use PCA for this discomfort.

Hypotension
Opioids themselves do not usually cause hypotension, but may unmask an existing hypovolemia.

ALTERNATIVE ROUTES

SUBCUTANEOUS PCA
Although the onset of analgesia will be slower, the subcutaneous route can also be used for PCA. This may be indicated if another drug that is incompatible with morphine is running in the primary IV line or if there is no IV access. Two suggestions for management of subcutaneous PCA are outlined below.

1. The same drug and same drug concentration as for IV PCA can be used but the following changes to the PCA program are suggested:
   - double the bolus dose
   - double the lock-out interval to 10 minutes
   - where possible, increase the dose duration to 5 minutes

   Because the bolus dose is given over 5 minutes and the drug is diluted, it is usually possible to administer meperidine (pethidine), as well as morphine and hydromorphone, by this route.

2. An alternative approach to subcutaneous PCA is as follows:
   - increase the concentration by a factor of 5 (to reduce the volume infused into the subcutaneous tissue)
   - increase the size of the bolus dose
   - use the same lock-out interval as for the IV route
   - use a continuous background infusion if there are clinical indications

Epidural PCA

The epidural route can also be used for I
commonly used for acute pain manageme
units. For further details see Chapter 6.

THE OPIOID-TOLERANT PATIENT

Opioid-tolerant patients can be divided into two groups: patients with an addiction to opioids, and those receiving opioids for the long-term treatment of chronic or cancer pain. The use of PCA can often be successful in these patients as they are likely to be tolerant to opioids (for definitions of tolerance, dependence and addiction see Chapter 1) and require higher than average doses. The easiest way to achieve this is to allow these patients to titrate their own analgesia.

Patients with an addiction to opioids

Addiction was initially believed to be a contraindication to the use of PCA. However, PCA is now recognized as a potentially useful method of providing pain relief in these patients, partly because of their often large opioid requirements and partly because it helps to avoid staff/patient confrontations about pain relief.

General management

The aims of treatment in this group of patients are twofold: to provide good pain relief and to prevent signs and symptoms of withdrawal. It is important to outline the treatment plans from the start. The patient should be assured that staff will aim for good analgesia but that the onset of sedation may prevent further increases in dose. These patients can have quite unrealistic expectations of pain relief and typically report high pain scores even in the presence of marked sedation.

Management contracts need to be established that include expected duration of treatment, plans for dose reductions (a gradual dose reduction may not occur spontaneously) and the choice of drugs available (meperidine should not be used as doses are likely to exceed 1000 mg and readily lead to the development

meperidine toxicity). The dangers associated with tamper-
with equipment or the use of illicit drugs in addition to PCA
should be explained. Management plans should be agreed to and
adhered to by all medical and nursing staff involved in the treatment of the patient.

If the patient is not in an addiction treatment program, the
immediate postoperative or post-injury period is not the time to
discuss the various options available. It is better to gain the
confidence of the patient by providing good analgesia and leave
any discussion about the treatment of addiction until later.

It is not uncommon for patients addicted to opioids to be
addicted to other drugs (e.g. alcohol, barbiturates or benzodiazepines), and signs and symptoms of withdrawal from these drugs
need to be monitored. Drug and alcohol rehabilitation services
should be involved in the treatment of these patients.

Management of PCA

Larger than average bolus doses will often be needed and there is a
clinical impression that these patients benefit from the addition of
a continuous (background) infusion. If the patient is in a methadone treatment program, the daily methadone dose can be used to
estimate the rate of the continuous infusion. If not, the rate can be
based on the size of the bolus dose required (rate in mg per hour =
bolus dose in mg).

Once the patient is tolerating unlimited oral fluids, oral analgesia can be commenced. If the patient is in a methadone treatment
program, methadone can be restarted at the normal maintenance
dose and additional oral analgesia (e.g. oxycodone) ordered
according to prior PCA opioid requirements. High PCA dose
requirements may mean that there is a delay before the patient
can be managed with oral opioids alone.

PATIENTS WITH CHRONIC OR CANCER PAIN

Patients requiring opioids for the long-term treatment of pain are
also likely to be tolerant to the drugs and require larger than
average doses. As with those patients with an addiction to
opioids, PCA can often be successfully used to treat acute pain.
Bolus doses may need to be larger than average and the addition

of a continuous (background) infusion is often helpful. The rates for this infusion can be based on the dose of any opioid the patient is already taking. In these patients too, meperidine should not be used.

Although this group of patients will not have the same psychological dependence on opioids as those with an addiction to the drugs, there may well be significant psychological factors that need to be taken into account in the treatment of their acute pain. Chronic pain may alter the perception to any new pain; the ability to cope with any new pain may depend on the significance attached to it. Acute pain may, for example, signify an exacerbation or progression of the disease; an operation may be expected to cure the pain or may only be an additional source of pain; or the operation may be a palliative procedure, reminding the patient of their limited life expectancy.

If an operation (or other intervention) is expected to cure the pain, the patient will no longer require long-term opioid therapy. To avoid any symptoms of withdrawal in patients who have been taking opioids for a prolonged period (as little as 7–10 days), the drugs should not be abruptly discontinued in the postoperative period. Instead, the total daily dose should be reduced by 20–25% each day.

Sometimes the pain may not be responsive to opioids, as is the case with neuropathic pain, and other drugs or interventional methods of pain relief may be needed.

Chronic pain is a complex interaction of many elements including not only the pain stimulus but also behavioral, psychological and other factors. Assistance from other services, including pain clinics, palliative care and psychiatric services, may be needed.

REFERENCES AND FURTHER READING

Eige S. (1992) PCA opioids: common side effects and their treatment. In *Acute Pain – Mechanisms and Management* (eds Sinatra R.S., Hord A.H., Ginsberg B. and Preble L.M.). Mosby Year Book, St Louis.

Ferrante F.M., Ostheimer G.W. and Covino B.G. (eds) (1990) *Patient-controlled Analgesia.* Blackwell Scientific Publications, Cambridge, Mass.

Gil K.M., Ginsberg B., Muir M., Sykes D. and Williams D.A. (1990) Patient-controlled analgesia in postoperative pain: the relation of psychological factors to pain and analgesic use. *Clinical Journal of Pain* **6**, 137–142.

Owen H., Plummer J.L., Armstrong I., Mather L.E. and Cousins M.J.C. (1989) Variables of patient-controlled analgesia: 1. Bolus size. *Anaesthesia* **44**, 7–10.

Owen H., Szekely S.M., Plummer J.L., Cushnie J.M. and Mather L.E. (1989) Variables of patient-controlled analgesia: 2. Concurrent infusion. *Anaesthesia* **44**, 11–13.

Parker R.K., Holtman B. and White P.F. (1993) Effects of a nighttime opioid infusion with PCA therapy on patient comfort and analgesic requirements after abdominal hysterectomy. *Anesthesiology* **76**, 362–367.

Ready L.B., Ashburn M., Caplan R.A., Carr D.B., Connis R.T., Dixon C.L., Hubbard L. and Rice L.J. (1995) Practice Guidelines for Acute Pain Management in the Perioperative Setting – a report of the American Society of Anesthesiologists Task Force on Pain Management, Acute Pain Section. *Anesthesiology* **82**, 1071–1081.

Sechzer P.H. (1968) Objective measurement of pain. *Anesthesiology* **29**, 209–210.

APPENDIX

Examples of acute pain management flowsheets and standard orders for patient-controlled analgesia, reproduced with permission of the Acute Pain Services at the Royal Adelaide Hospital, Adelaide, Australia and the University of Washington Medical Center, Seattle, Wash., USA.

5A Royal Adelaide Hospital chart for observations and record of drug administration.

5B University of Washington pain management flowsheet.

5C University of Washington intravenous PCA physician order sheet.

5D Royal Adelaide Hospital Acute Pain Service PCA standard orders.

5E University of Washington primary care service intravenous PCA physician orders.

APPENDIX 5A

	ROYAL ADELAIDE HOSPITAL

ACUTE PAIN SERVICE
SPECIAL OBSERVATIONS
AND RECORD OF DRUG
ADMINISTRATION

Unit Record No.: _____

Surname: _____

Given Names: _____

Date of Birth: _____ Sex: _____

Date/Time	Drug	Dose	Pain score .... X 0 2 4 6 8 10/S	Sed'n	Resp	PR	BP	Comments	Signature MO or RN

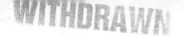

APPENDIX 5A

ADVERSE DRUG REACTIONS				
Drug	Date	Details		Signature

PAIN SCORE: 0 = no pain 10 = worst pain imaginable

SEDATION SCORE:
0 = none
1 = mild, occasionally drowsy, easy to rouse
2 = moderate, constantly drowsy, easy to rouse
3 = severe, somnolent, difficult to rouse
S = normally asleep, easy to rouse

Date/ Time	Drug	Dose	Pain score .... X 0 2 4 6 8 10/S	Sed'n	Resp	PR	BP	Comments	Signature MO or RN

APPENDIX 5B

SEDATION SCALE
0 = None
1 = Mild
    (occasionally drowsy; easy to arouse)
2 = Moderate
    (frequently drowsy; easy to arouse)
3 = Severe
    (somnolent; difficult to arouse)
S = Normal sleep
    (easy to arouse)

ANALGESIA SCALE
0 = no pain
10 = worst pain imaginable

MONITORING
PCA: Q ___ hr x ___ hrs;
     then Q ___ hrs

EPIDURAL:
     Q ___ hr x ___ hrs;
     then Q ___ hrs

Date																	
Time																	
Resp. Rate																	
Sedation																	
Analgesia																	

PATIENT CONTROLLED ANALGESIA

Med (mg/ml)																	
Incremental Dose																	
Lockout Interval																	
4 Hour Limit																	
Bolus Dose																	
Continuous Infusion																	
Cumulative Dose																	
Clear volume																	
Syringe added																	

EPIDURAL																
PF Morphine																
Fentanyl																
Continuous Infusion																
Initials																
Signature	Signature					Signature						Signature				

UNIVERSITY OF WASHINGTON MEDICAL CENTERS
HARBORVIEW MEDICAL CENTER
UNIVERSITY OF WASHINGTON MEDICAL CENTER
SEATTLE, WASHINGTON

PAIN MANAGEMENT FLOWSHEET

UH 0827   SEP 89

APPENDIX 5C

1. PCA PRESCRIPTION:

MODE:	☐ PCA Only	☐ PCA + Continuous Infusion		☐ Continuous Infusion only
DRUG:	☐ Morphine 1 mg / ml	☐ Meperidine 10 mg / ml	☐ Hydromorphone 0.2 mg / ml	☐ Other: _____ mg - mcg / ml
PCA MODE: Incremental Dose	_____ mg	_____ mg	_____ mg	_____ mg - mcg
Lockout	8 minutes	8 minutes	8 minutes	_____ minutes
4 Hour Limit	30 mg	300 mg	6 mg	_____ mg - mcg
OPTIONAL INFUSION MODE: (Recommended starting rate)	_____ mg/hr (0.5 mg/hr)	_____ mg/hr (5 mg/hr)	_____ mg/hr (0.1 mg/hr)	_____ mg - mcg/hr (Consult APS)
Instructions for infusion:	☐ Continuous ☐ Infuse from 2200 to 0600 nightly	☐ Continuous ☐ Infuse from 2200 to 0600 nightly	☐ Continuous ☐ Infuse from 2200 to 0600 nightly	☐ Continuous ☐ Infuse from 2200 to 0600 nightly
LOADING DOSES: (via PCA pump when block recedes or for breakthrough pain)	_____ mg q 5 min to a maximum of _____ mg	_____ mg q 5 min to a maximum of _____ mg	_____ mg q 5 min to a maximum of _____ mg	_____ mg/mcg q 5 min to a maximum of _____ mg/mcg
FOR INADEQUATE RELIEF: after 1 hr with initial pump settings:	Increase Incremental Dose to _____ mg	Increase Incremental Dose to _____ mg	Increase Incremental Dose to _____ mg	Increase Incremental Dose to _____ mg/mcg
FOR INADEQUATE RELIEF: after 1 additional hr:	Decrease lockout to _____ min	Decrease lockout to _____ min	Decrease lockout to _____ min	Decrease lockout to _____ min

2. **No systemic narcotics or other CNS depressants** to be given except as ordered by the Acute Pain Service (APS).

3. **PCA not to be discontinued except by Acute Pain Service.**

4. **MONITORING:** Respiratory rate, analgesic level, sedation scale - q 2 h for 8 hours; then q 4 h while patient is on PCA. Document on "Pain Management Flowsheet."

5. **TREATMENT OF SIDE EFFECTS:**

   A. Call APS for sedation scale = 3, RR < 8 per minute, or pCO_2 > 50 mmHg.

   B. NALOXONE 0.1 - 0.4 mg, IV <u>stat</u> for sedation scale > 3 plus RR < 8 per minute. Call APS.

   C. METOCLOPRAMIDE 10 mg IV q 4 h prn for nausea / vomiting. In addition, if age < 60 years, TRANSDERMAL SCOPOLAMINE PATCH to either mastoid area. Change q 72 h prn.

   D. DIPHENHYDRAMINE 25 mg, IV or PO q 6 h for severe itching.

   E. For urinary retention, "in and out" catheter, prn.

6. If age < 60 years, TRIAZOLAM 0.125 mg q h s prn. MR x 1.

7. For inadequate analgesia or other problems related to PCA, call the Acute Pain Service.

Dr. _____ on the Acute Pain Service was notified about this patient at _____ hours.

_____ M. D.

DATE	TIME	PHYSICIAN

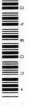

UNIVERSITY OF WASHINGTON MEDICAL CENTERS
HARBORVIEW MEDICAL CENTER · UW MEDICAL CENTER
SEATTLE, WASHINGTON

**ACUTE PAIN SERVICE INTRAVENOUS PATIENT
CONTROLLED ANALGESIA (PCA) PHYSICIAN ORDERS**

UH N 0840 REV FEB 94

WHITE · MEDICAL RECORD
CANARY · PHARMACY
PINK · NURSING

UR 72.2

ROYAL ADELAIDE HOSPITAL

ACUTE PAIN SERVICE
PATIENT CONTROLLED
ANALGESIA (PCA)
Standard Orders

Unit Record No.: _____

Surname: _____

Given Names: _____

Date of Birth: _____   Sex: _____

1. No systemic opioids or sedatives to be given except as ordered by the APS.
2. Naloxone 400 micrograms at bedside.
3. Oxygen at .... 1/min via nasal specs or .... mask.
4. One-way "antireflux" valve to be used in line at all times.
5. **Monitoring and documentation:**
   a) Record pain score, sedation score and respiratory rate <u>hourly for 8 hours and then 2 hourly.</u>
      Omit pain score if asleep.
   b) Record current dose "since reset" at each monitoring interval. When the syringe is changed,
      check the machine settings, reset the PCA and record "total dose since reset".
6. For inadequate analgesia or other problems related to PCA, page the rostered APS anaesthetist. After
   1730 hours this will be the 2nd on-call ESS anaesthetic registrar.

7. **PCA OPIOID ORDER:**

   a) Drug ....   Route if other than IV ....

   b) <u>PCA machine settings</u>

      * loading dose = 0 (loading dose to be given in Recovery or by APS staff)

      * bolus dose = ... mg   * dose duration = "stat"

* lockout duration = 5 minutes   * concentration = ... mg/ml

* background infusion = ... mg (= .... ml) /hr

c) If pain not controlled after 1 hour, increase bolus dose to .... mg.

d) **If sedation score = 2, reduce size of bolus dose by half and cease any background infusion.**

e) Cease PCA if patient becomes confused.

8. **TREATMENT OF SIDE EFFECTS:**

a) **Respiratory depression.**

If sedation score = 3 OR respiratory rate less than 8/min AND sedation score = 2 or 3, give 100 micrograms NALOXONE IV stat. Repeat PRN up to a total of 400 micrograms. Cease PCA and call APS.

b) **Nausea/vomiting.**

Give METOCLOPRAMIDE 10mg IV 4 hourly PRN. If metoclopramide ineffective, give DROPERIDOL 250 micrograms IV 6 hourly PRN.

(5 mg droperidol [= 1ml] made up to 20 ml with saline = 250 micrograms/ml)

9. **SIGNATURE OF ANAESTHETIST** .... DATE ....

(Print name ....) TIME ....

10. Cease above orders

Signature .... Date .... Time ....

APPENDIX 5E

PRIMARY CARE SERVICE INTRAVENOUS
PATIENT CONTROLLED ANALGESIA (PCA) PHYSICIAN ORDERS

1. PCA PRESCRIPTION

DRUG: (check one)	☐ Morphine 1 mg/ml	☐ Meperidine 10 mg/ml	☐ Hydromorphone 0.2 mg/ml
PCA MODE:			
Incremental dose (range)	_____ mg (0.5 - 1 mg)	_____ mg (5 - 10 mg)	_____ mg (0.1 - 0.3 mg)
Lockout	8 minutes	8 minutes	8 minutes
4 Hour Limit	30 mg	300 mg	6 mg
	<u>Caution</u>: 24 h limit = 100 mg	<u>Caution</u>: 24 h limit = 1000 mg	<u>Caution</u>: 24 h limit = 15 mg
OPTIONAL LOADING DOSES (If necesary on initiation of therapy, give boluses from PCA pump)	2X the current incremental dose q 5 min up to a maximum of 5 doses		
FOR INADEQUATE PAIN RELIEF (After 1 hour with initial pump settings)	Increase initial incremental dose by 50%		
FOR INADEQUATE PAIN RELIEF (After 1 additional hour)	Decrease lockout to 6 min		

FOR INCIDENT OR BREAKTHROUGH PAIN
(Give boluses from PCA pump)

2X the current incremental dose q 5 min up to a maximum of 5 doses per event

INFUSION MODE

Caution: use only when PCA mode alone proves inadequate.

Check one of the boxes to initiate:

☐ 2200 - 0600 h
☐ continuous

Rate: mg/h equal to current incremental dose.

2. **AVOID CONCURRENT USE OF OTHER OPIOIDS AND/OR CNS DEPRESSANTS.**

3. **MONITORING:** Respiratory rate, analgesic level, and sedation scale - q2h for 8 hours, then q4h while patient is on PCA. Document on "Pain Management Flowsheet."

4. **TREATMENT OF SIDE EFFECTS:**
   A. Call physician for sedation scale = 2, RR<8 per minute, or pCO_2 >50 mmHg.
   B. NALOXONE 0.1 - 0.4mg, IV stat for sedation scale =3 plus RR <8/minute. Call physician.
   C. METOCLOPRAMIDE 10 mg IV q4h prn for nausea/vomiting. In addition, if age <60 years, TRANSDERMAL SCOPOLAMINE PATCH to either mastoid area. Change q72h prn.
   D. DIPHENHYDRAMINE, 25 mg, IV or PO q6h for severe itching.
   E. For urinary retention, "in and out" catheter, prn.

5. **ALTERNATIVE TREATMENT OF SIDE EFFECTS:** _____

6. **FOR SLEEP:** _____

7. **FOR INADEQUATE ANALGESIA OR OTHER PROBLEMS RELATED TO PCA:**
   Call physician @ pager # _____

Date	Time	Physician	M.D.

CHAPTER 6

EPIDURAL AND INTRATHECAL ANALGESIA

Development;

Anatomy;

Contraindications;

Drugs used for epidural analgesia;

Drugs used for intrathecal analgesia;

Monitoring;

Standard orders and nursing

policies and protocols;

Daily management;

Subsequent analgesic regimens;

Complications;

Patient-controlled epidural analgesia

Epidural and intrathecal analgesia are specialized techniques of pain relief that will be initiated by an anesthesiologist (if used after spinal surgery an epidural catheter may be placed by the surgeon at the end of the operation) and an anesthesiologist will be responsible for their continuing management. Nevertheless, junior medical staff must have an understanding of these forms of analgesia so that they are aware of possible complications and drug interactions. In addition, they are likely to be asked about these methods of pain relief by patients and their relatives.

With careful patient selection, frequent monitoring, appropriate standard orders and nursing policies and procedures, extensive nursing education, and delegation of all responsibility for pain relief to one group of specialist medical staff (anesthesiologists), epidural and intrathecal analgesia can be safely managed on general hospital wards.

DEVELOPMENT

Epidural analgesia using local anesthetic agents for up to 5 days was first used for the treatment of postoperative pain in 1949. The technique gained in popularity, especially in obstetric units for analgesia during labor, but use outside these units was limited.

Intrathecal morphine was first used for the treatment of back pain by Dr Katawata in Japan, in 1901. Although excellent pain relief was reported, the technique was not used again for another 75 years. In the mid-1970s opioid receptors were identified in the brain and spinal cord; in 1976 it was recognized that spinal opioids were capable of producing analgesia in animals; in 1979 epidural and intrathecal opioids were again used to provide analgesia in humans. The progression from preliminary observation to widespread clinical use has been rapid, especially following the relatively recent, more organized approach to acute pain management and the introduction of acute pain services.

Epidural and intrathecal analgesia (opioids alone or a mixture of opioid and local anesthetic) can provide better pain relief than other methods of opioid administration, and are more likely to lead to a reduction in postoperative morbidity, particularly in the high risk patient. The risk of complications is very small but must always be weighed against possible advantages.

ANATOMY

The spinal cord and brain are covered by three membranes called meninges: the outer layer is called the dura mater; the middle layer, the arachnoid, lies just below the dura and both form the dural sac; the inner layer, the pia mater, adheres to the surface of the cord and the brain. The *epidural space* lies between the dura mater and the bone and ligaments of the spinal canal (**Figure**

6.1). It is only a potential space and contains blood vessels, nerve roots, fat and connective tissue. Deep to the arachnoid membrane is the subarachnoid or *intrathecal space*, containing cerebrospinal fluid (CSF) and the spinal cord above the level of L1-2 or the cauda equina (the lumbar and sacral nerve roots) below L1-2. The dural sac ends at S2.

To obtain *epidural analgesia*, analgesic drugs are administered directly into the epidural space. An epidural catheter is usually placed to enable repeated doses or an infusion of the drug to be given. Drugs administered directly into the CSF and used for *intrathecal analgesia* are more commonly given as a single dose through a spinal needle at the time of spinal anesthesia. The

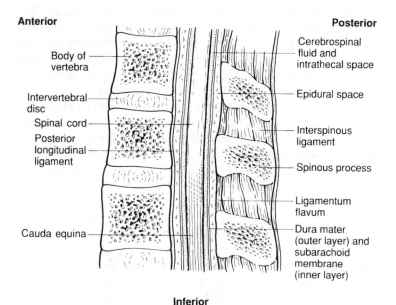

Superior

Anterior · Posterior

Body of vertebra

Cerebrospinal fluid and intrathecal space

Intervertebral disc

Epidural space

Spinal cord

Posterior longitudinal ligament

Interspinous ligament

Spinous process

Ligamentum flavum

Cauda equina

Dura mater (outer layer) and subarachoid membrane (inner layer)

Inferior

Figure 6.1
Anatomy of the spinal cord

doses of drugs required for intrathecal analgesia are much smaller than those required for epidural analgesia.

CONTRAINDICATIONS

UNTRAINED NURSING AND MEDICAL STAFF

Epidural and intrathecal analgesia should only be used in hospital wards where staff have received specific teaching about these methods of pain relief. The staff should have a good understanding of the techniques and the monitoring requirements and be able to recognize and treat (according to written orders) inadequate analgesia and side effects. Many institutions require some form of 'accreditation' before nurses are allowed to take responsibility for patients with epidural or intrathecal analgesia, especially if they are required to administer bolus doses of the drugs. In addition, these methods of pain relief should only be used when an anesthesiologist is available to review patients daily and whenever problems arise.

PATIENT REJECTION

For many reasons patients may not want epidural or intrathecal analgesia; for example, they may have heard of possible complications, either from friends or from the media. A full explanation needs to be given to each patient and the risks and possible benefits explained.

CONTRAINDICATIONS TO THE PLACEMENT OF AN EPIDURAL OR SPINAL NEEDLE OR CATHETER

There are a number of reasons why placement of a needle or catheter may be contraindicated, or at least relatively contraindicated (that is the potential benefits of placement must outweigh possible risks): local or generalized sepsis may lead to an infection of the epidural space; coagulation disorders or concurrent medication with anticoagulant drugs may increase the risk of an epidural hematoma; epidural or intrathecal analgesia may be implicated in any progression of central nervous system diseases such as multiple sclerosis; and profound hypotension may occur in a hypovolemic patient. All of these problems can arise spontaneously, but insertion of an epidural or intrathecal needle or catheter may increase the risk of them occurring. If the dura has been punctured, either inadvertently during insertion of an epidural catheter or during spinal surgery, part of any drug injected into the epidural space may gain direct access to the CSF. The patient must be observed very closely if a decision is made to proceed with epidural analgesia.

In general, the insertion of epidural or intrathecal needles and catheters is avoided in patients who are fully anticoagulated. For patients on low-dose subcutaneous heparin therapy, avoidance of catheter placement within 4–6 hours after the last dose is suggested. Postoperative anticoagulation with either warfarin or heparin means that care also needs to be taken with the timing of the removal of an epidural or intrathecal catheter. In general, it is probably wise to remove catheters before full anticoagulation with warfarin (1–2 days); no sooner than 1–2 hours after cessation of a heparin infusion; and 4–6 hours after a dose of subcutaneous heparin. Intraoperative heparinization may be required for some operations and it is suggested that epidural and spinal needles and catheters be placed at least 1 hour before the heparin is given.

The contraindications to epidural and intrathecal analgesia are summarized in **Box 6.1**.

▼

Possible contraindications to epidural and intrathecal analgesia

Untrained staff
Patient rejection
Contraindications to catheter or needle placement
    local or general sepsis
    coagulation disorders or treatment with anticoagulant medications
    some central or spinal neurological diseases
    hypovolemia
Presence of a dural puncture

Box 6.1

DRUGS USED FOR EPIDURAL ANALGESIA

Two classes of drugs are commonly used for epidural analgesia: opioids and local anesthetics. They can be given as repeated bolus doses (usually morphine, diamorphine or meperidine) or by infusion (any of the opioids or, frequently, a combination of opioid and local anesthetic). All drugs given either epidurally or intrathecally should be preservative-free. The doses and infusion rates suggested are guidelines only and may vary according to patient age, medical condition, site of injection and other factors.

OPIOID DRUGS

Site of action
When an opioid is injected into the epidural space, part of the dose crosses the dura and arachnoid membrane and enters the CSF; part is absorbed into epidural veins and enters the systemic circulation; and part binds to epidural fat.

From the CSF a proportion of the drug is taken up into the spinal cord and reaches opioid receptors in the dorsal column. The more lipid-soluble the drug, the more rapid the onset of analgesia but the shorter the duration of action. The quicker onset is because transfer across the dura and uptake to receptor sites in the spinal cord is more rapid than with the less lipid-soluble opioids such as morphine. The shorter duration of action results from faster removal from receptor sites through spinal cord blood flow.

Bulk flow of CSF in a rostral direction means that any drug remaining in the CSF will be carried to opioid receptors further from the site of injection. The less lipid-soluble drugs, such as morphine, are cleared less rapidly from the CSF (that is, uptake into nervous tissue and blood vessels is slower) and are more likely to have a greater degree of spread. For example, lumbar epidural morphine can be used for pain relief following thoracic operations, but lumbar epidural administration of fentanyl will not be as effective for the same operation (i.e. the effectiveness of the lipid-soluble opioids is much more dependent on the site of injection than is the case with drugs such as morphine). Meperidine (pethidine) is of intermediate lipid solubility, therefore the degree of spread of meperidine in CSF is intermediate between morphine and fentanyl.

Rostral spread of drug in the CSF also has potential disadvantages as respiratory depression may occur if sufficient drug remains in the CSF when it reaches the brain stem and the respiratory center. Rostral spread of drug can also contribute to the development of other side effects such as nausea, vomiting and pruritus.

The proportion of epidurally administered opioid that is absorbed into the systemic circulation will contribute to analgesia and the development of opioid-related side effects. The more lipid-soluble the opioid, the greater the proportion of any dose that will be absorbed systemically.

Doses

The analgesic efficacy of morphine is greater when given epidurally compared with parenteral administration; that is, a much smaller dose is needed to achieve the same or better degree of pain relief. The more lipid-soluble the opioid, the greater the systemic uptake and the less the difference between the epidural and parenteral doses needed to provide the same level of analgesia.

For the longer-acting opioids, administration by infusion offers little or no advantage over intermittent bolus doses in terms of analgesic efficacy. In addition, unlike PCA machines, there is no restriction to the access of opioids (by staff or patients) delivered by most infusion or syringe pumps. However, the use of an infusion may reduce the incidence of side effects and will decrease the number of times the catheter and filter are handled. This will reduce the risk of a break in sterile technique and therefore reduce the risk of infection. The highly lipid-soluble opioids, fentanyl and sufentanil, are best administered by continuous infusion because of their short duration of action.

Commonly used drugs, doses, approximate rates of onset and durations of action, and infusion rates are listed in **Box 6.2**. The quicker onset of a drug such as fentanyl can be useful in the event of breakthrough pain in a patient receiving epidural morphine, when it can be administered in addition to another dose of morphine so that rapid pain relief can be achieved. The short duration of action of meperidine (pethidine) means that bolus doses may have to be given every 1–2 hours. It is possible, therefore, if large total doses are required, for a patient to develop normeperidine (norpethidine) toxicity (see Chapter 2).

The total dose of opioid administered into the epidural space is the primary determinant of analgesic activity but the volume in which the dose is administered may help to determine the spread of the dose. This is particularly so for the more lipid-soluble opioids such as fentanyl and sufentanil.

As with any opioid, regardless of route, the initial dose should be based on the age of the patient and subsequent doses titrated to effect. Morphine is commonly used when opioids alone are administered for epidural analgesia. Suggested initial doses via lumbar catheters for non-thoracic surgery or via thoracic catheters for thoracic surgery range from 4 mg in patients less than 45 years old to 1 mg in patients over 75 years old.

Epidural opioids:
Commonly used bolus doses and infusion rates[a]

Opioid	Bolus (mg)	Onset (min)	Duration[b] (hr)	Infusion (mg/hr)	Lipid solubility[c]
Morphine	1–6	30–60	6–24	0.1–0.75	1
Hydromorphone	1–2	10–15	6–16	0.1–0.4	1
Diamorphine	2–6	5–10	6–12	0.2–0.8	10
Meperidine (pethidine)	20–50	5–10	1–6	10–30	30
Fentanyl	0.025–0.1	5–10	1–4	0.025–0.1	800
Sufentanil	0.01–0.05	5–10	1–4	0.01–0.05	1500

[a] effective doses will vary depending on patient age, medical condition and site of injection
[b] duration of analgesia varies widely; higher doses will have a longer duration of action
[c] octanol/pH 7.4 buffer partition coefficient relative to morphine
Table compiled from values obtained from listed references

Box 6.2

Side effects

Cardiovascular system Hypotension is unlikely following epidural administration of opioids unless the patient is already hypovolemic. It has, however, been reported (rarely) following the use of meperidine, and this may be in part due to the fact that this drug has some intrinsic local anesthetic activity.

Respiratory system Respiratory depression is a possible complication of epidural opioids and may occur at two different intervals:

- *Early* – usually within 2 hours of injection, may occur if high blood levels of opioid follow absorption of drug from the epidural space into the systemic circulation.
- *Delayed* – which may not be seen for over 6–12 hours after the opioid was given, results from the rostral migration of drug in the CSF to the brain stem and respiratory center. The onset is usually gradual with the patient becoming progressively more sedated. If delayed respiratory depression does occur it can persist for many hours. It is less likely with more lipid-soluble drugs – e.g. meperidine and fentanyl – as these drugs, once in the CSF, are subject to rapid uptake into spinal cord tissue and blood vessels. The risk of significant concentrations of these drugs reaching the respiratory center due to rostral spread in the CSF is therefore much less.

There is an increased risk of respiratory depression associated with:

- increasing patient age
- high doses of epidural (or intrathecal) opioid
- the opioid-naive patient
- concurrent use of sedatives or systemic opioids (including long-acting sedatives or large doses of parenteral opioids given before or during an operation)

As with other methods of opioid administration, a decrease in respiratory rate can be a late and unreliable sign of respiratory depression and, therefore, frequent assessments of patient sedation should also be made. If a patient becomes excessively sedated, subsequent bolus doses should be reduced and infusions stopped or decreased. Naloxone may be required (see **Box 6.11**).

Motor function Epidural opioids will not affect motor function.

Central nervous system Sedation, nausea and vomiting can occur after the epidural administration of opioids. In part these side effects may result from absorption of drug into the systemic circulation; they can also be due to rostral spread of the drug in the CSF, in which case they are more likely to occur some hours after administration of the opioid.

Antiemetics should be administered and consideration given to reducing the dose of opioid. It is important to remember that postoperative nausea and vomiting is multifactorial and conditions or drugs other than the opioids may be responsible. Severe and intractable nausea and vomiting may respond to opioid antagonists or agonist-antagonists (see Chapter 2).

Pruritus Pruritus, particularly over the face, chest and abdomen, is more likely to follow the epidural (and intrathecal) administration of opioids, especially morphine, than administration by any other route. It appears to be less common in the older patient. Although the exact mechanism is unknown, it is presumed to be centrally mediated and a consequence of activation of µ receptors in the spinal cord. Small doses or an infusion of an opioid antagonist or agonist-antagonist can be used to treat the pruritus without reversing the analgesia. More recently, small doses of an anesthetic induction agent, propofol, have been observed to relieve pruritus following epidural morphine. Antihistamines may be effective in some cases, even though histamine release plays a negligible role in the development of pruritus. However, the sedative effects of these drugs may increase the risk of respiratory depression.

There are other causes of itching. For example, the plastic covering of a mattress may result in sweating and itching of the back; itching may occur under dressings or plaster casts.

Urinary retention Urinary retention is a possible complication of epidural opioids and is due to inhibition of the micturition reflex evoked by increases in bladder volume. However, it is not inevitable and does not require routine prophylactic catheterization of all patients. If retention does occur, small doses of an opioid antagonist or agonist-antagonist may be given. If this is unsuccessful, a urinary catheter will be needed, but it can be 'in-out' and does not have to remain in situ.

Gastrointestinal system Epidural opioids decrease bowel motility but to a lesser degree than equianalgesic doses of opioid given by other routes.

LOCAL ANESTHETIC DRUGS

Site of action
Epidurally administered local anesthetic drugs gain access to the nerve roots and spinal cord by crossing the dura and subarachnoid membranes. Part of any given dose will be, as for opioids, absorbed into the systemic circulation.

Doses
While often used to provide analgesia and anesthesia during surgery, local anesthetic drugs are rarely used as the sole agent for epidural analgesia in general wards. An infusion of a combination with opioids is, however, common and doses and infusion rates are discussed in the next section.

Side effects
Local neurotoxicity or systemic toxicity (from an excessive dose or from an otherwise safe dose inadvertently injected into a blood vessel) may follow the epidural administration of local anesthetic solutions (for details refer to Chapter 2). Blockade of autonomic and motor fibres as well as sensory nerves (also see Chapter 2) may result in other side effects, including the following.

Cardiovascular system Sympathetic block can lead to hypotension. The greater the number of segments blocked and the higher the concentration and total dose of epidural local anesthetic, the more likely a decrease in blood pressure is to occur. In the low concentrations usually used in combination with opioids for pain relief on general wards, significant hypotension is unlikely unless the patient is also hypovolemic. However, even partial sympathetic blockade may prevent compensatory mechanisms, which usually prevent venous pooling when the patient sits or stands, from being fully effective and postural or orthostatic hypotension is therefore possible. If the block extends above T4 (nipple line) and sufficient concentration of local anesthetic agent is used, the cardioaccelerator fibers to the heart may be blocked leading to bradycardia.

If hypotension occurs it will normally respond to intravenous fluids but vasopressors (such as ephedrine) may be required. These should be available in all wards where epidural local anesthetic drugs or local anesthetic/opioid mixtures are used. Bradycardia may respond to atropine, although if bradycardia or hypotension are severe, epinephrine (adrenaline) may be more effective.

Respiratory system The diaphragm, supplied by cervical nerves 3 to 5, is the most important muscle of involuntary respiration. Therefore, epidural local anesthetics in normal doses are very unlikely to impair normal respiration significantly. Motor block of intercostal muscles can, however, reduce a patient's ability to take a deep breath and cough. Patients with pulmonary disease may be unable to tolerate a block of their intercostal muscles.

Motor/sensory block Depending on the concentration of local anesthetic agent and the total dose used, other sensory nerves and motor nerves may be blocked. Immobility is not desirable after injury or surgery, so low concentrations of local anesthetic are often used for the treatment of acute pain in general wards in an attempt to preferentially block smaller sensory fibers while avoiding a block of the larger motor fibers (*differential block* – see Chapter 2).

The low concentrations of local anesthetic drugs are often given in combination with an opioid and by continuous infusion (see below). Using this combination, good analgesia can be achieved with a minimum of motor block or block of other sensory nerves. If a patient complains of numbness or weakness, the infusion should be stopped for a short while and then restarted at a lower rate. If the problem persists the concentration of the local anesthetic solution can be reduced, or the technique changed to the use of an epidural opioid only. Numbness and weakness may also be the first signs of catheter migration into the CSF (very rare). Pressure areas have been reported following epidural analgesia, presumably due to a combination of immobility and decreased sensation.

Central nervous system Unless local anesthetic doses are large there is unlikely to be significant sedation or nausea and vomiting.

Pruritus Pruritus is not a side effect of epidural local anesthetic agents.

Urinary retention As with epidural opioids urinary retention can occur but is not inevitable and does not require routine prophylactic catheterization.

Gastrointestinal system Bowel motility is unimpaired or even improved, although addition of opioids to the local anesthetic solution will have the same effects as opioids alone.

COMBINATIONS OF LOCAL ANESTHETIC AND OPIOID DRUGS

The side effects of opioid and local anesthetic agents used in epidural analgesia are compared in **Box 6.3**.

In an attempt to minimize the adverse effects of each class of drug and provide better analgesia than that attained with either agent alone, a combination of an opioid and a low concentration of local anesthetic solution (colloquially called an 'epidural cocktail') is often given by continuous infusion. Studies comparing the analgesic efficacy of opioids alone with a combination of the two classes of drug do not always show a difference in pain relief at rest. However, if pain is assessed during movement, e.g. mobilization or coughing, the combination of opioid and local anesthetic solution results in better analgesia.

While the aim of the combination therapy is to obtain the full benefits of each class of drug before side effects from either class occur, little work has been done on the ideal ratio for each drug in the solution. A reasonable ratio for bupivacaine and fentanyl

Comparison of the side effects of opioid and local anesthetic epidural analgesia

	Opioid	Local anesthetic
Respiratory	Delayed depression Early depression	Usually unimpaired
Cardiovascular	Usually no reduction in blood pressure	Overt or postural hypotension Reduced heart rate with high block
Sedation	Yes	Mild/absent
Nausea/vomiting	Yes	Less common
Pruritus	Yes (give naloxone)	No
Motor	No effect	Block
Urinary retention	Yes	Yes
Gastrointestinal	Decreased motility	Increased motility

Adapted from Cousins and Mather (1984)

Box 6.3

seems to be 1 mg bupivacaine to about 4–5 µg fentanyl. The following are examples of commonly used mixtures:

- 0.0625% bupivacaine and 2 µg/ml fentanyl
- 0.08% bupivacaine and 4 µg/ml fentanyl
- 0.1% bupivacaine and 5 µg/ml fentanyl
- 0.125% bupivacaine and 5 µg/ml fentanyl

Combinations of bupivacaine and morphine (e.g. 0.1% bupivacaine and 0.025–0.1 mg/ml morphine), bupivacaine and meperidine (e.g. 0.1% bupivacaine and 1–2 mg/ml meperidine) and bupivacaine and diamorphine (0.1% bupivacaine and 0.05–0.1 mg/ml diamorphine) have also been used. It is the total dose of the drugs given that is important; the higher the concentration the lower the volume infused.

Local anesthetic drugs block nerve fibers at spinal segments immediately adjacent to their site of administration. The siting of the epidural catheter, in the middle of the dermatomal seg-ments to be covered, is therefore important when a combination of local anesthetic and opioid drugs is used.

Dose regimens

The infusion rates will vary according to the concentration of drugs in the solutions; the site of injury or operation (including the position relative to the site of epidural catheter placement); and the age of the patient. In institutions where nursing staff are allowed to administer 'top-up' doses as well as alter infusion rates, orders should include bolus doses of the solution for breakthrough pain. Suggested bolus doses and infusion rates for some of the combination solutions are listed in **Box 6.4**.

DRUGS USED FOR INTRATHECAL ANALGESIA

SITE OF ACTION

Opioids alone (i.e. not a combination of local anesthetic and opioid drugs) are commonly used for intrathecal analgesia. The opioid is delivered directly into the CSF, avoiding absorption by epidural fat and blood vessels. Because of rostral migration in the CSF, intrathecal opioids, particularly morphine, will spread to

---

▼ Suggestions for initial infusion rates and bolus doses using 0.0625–0.1% bupivacaine and 2–4 µg/ml fentanyl

	Younger patients	Older patients
Infusion rate (ml/hr)	8–15	4–10
PRN bolus doses (ml)	4–8	3–5

- Thoracic epidural infusions will, in general, require slightly smaller volumes than lumbar epidural infusions
- Lower infusion rates are needed if higher concentrations of drug are used

Box 6.4

receptors at higher levels in the spinal cord and may reach the brain stem.

DOSES

The doses of opioids administered intrathecally are much smaller than doses required for epidural analgesia but, as for epidural opioid analgesia, the more lipid-soluble the drug the more rapid the onset but shorter the duration of action.

All the drugs listed in **Box 6.5** have been used for intrathecal analgesia. Because meperidine (pethidine) has local anesthetic as well as opioid properties, it has been used as the sole spinal anesthetic agent (in larger doses of 30–50 mg) for a variety of lower limb operations.

Although most intrathecal opioids are given as a 'once only' dose at the time of spinal anesthesia, a catheter can be left in place. All spinal catheters must be clearly labelled to distinguish them from epidural catheters.

POSSIBLE SIDE EFFECTS

Side effects are similar to those that occur with epidural opioids. Although some believe that the incidence is higher with intrathecal opioids, this is, to a large extent, dose dependent.

With epidural opioids respiratory depression may occur owing to systemic absorption of the drug (early) or rostral spread of the

Intrathecal opioids			
Opioid	Dose (mg)	Onset (min)	Duration (hr)
Morphine	0.1–0.5	15–30	8–24
Meperidine (pethidine)	10–25	5–10	6–12
Fentanyl	0.006–0.02	5	2–4
Diamorphine	0.5–1	5	10–20

Table compiled from values obtained from listed references

Box 6.5

drug in the CSF to the respiratory center (delayed). If respiratory depression occurs following administration of intrathecal opioids, it will be delayed. As with epidural analgesia, it is less likely with the more lipid-soluble drugs. Increasing patient age, high doses of intrathecal opioid, an opioid-naive patient and concurrent use of sedatives or systemic opioids are associated with an increased risk of respiratory depression.

MONITORING

Pain score, sedation score and respiratory rate should be monitored at frequent intervals. Respiratory monitors that sound an alarm if ventilation is not detected and/or continuous pulse oximetry are used in some centers, especially for patients considered at higher risk of respiratory depression. However, these monitors should not be seen as a substitute for direct patient observation by well-trained nursing staff. If local anesthetic agents are used (alone or in combination with opioids), blood pressure and heart rate should also be recorded for at least the first 24 hours. Block height can be measured by testing the level at which the patient reports a change in sensation from cold to warmth when ice or alcohol is applied to the skin; however, the differences may not be very marked when low concentrations of local anesthetic are infused. The ability of a patient to raise a straight leg will provide evidence that lower extremity motor block is not excessive.

All observations should be documented (see examples of flowsheets in the appendix at the end of Chapter 5) at regular intervals (hourly for up to 24 hours and then every 2–4 hours is suggested), along with the total amount of drug delivered, the dose of any drug administered for the treatment of side effects and any changes that have been made to the infusion rates.

STANDARD ORDERS AND NURSING POLICIES AND PROTOCOLS

As for patient-controlled analgesia, standard orders and nursing policies and protocols are recommended to maximize the effectiveness of epidural and intrathecal analgesia and minimize the risk of complications. To reduce the risk of drugs or fluids intended for IV administration being inadvertently given via epidural or intrathecal catheters, all catheters should carry a clearly visible label.

STANDARD ORDERS

Standard orders need to cover a number of different areas, as follows.

Nondrug treatment orders

Nondrug treatment orders may include a statement to eliminate the concurrent ordering of CNS depressants or other opioids by others; orders for oxygen; availability of drugs to treat side effects; monitoring and documentation requirements; maintenance of IV access; and instructions as to whom to contact if problems occur.

Epidural or intrathecal drug orders

Orders for drug doses, infusion rates and instructions for the treatment of inadequate analgesia are required.

Orders for the treatment of side effects

The inclusion of standard orders for the recognition and management of side effects will minimize delays in treatment. To standardize the orders throughout the institution, preprinted forms are recommended. The important elements that should be included in these forms are listed in **Box 6.6**. The forms need to be completed and then signed and dated by the treating anesthesiologist.

Examples of preprinted epidural and intrathecal standard orders are included in the appendix at the end of this chapter.

Important elements of epidural analgesia preprinted orders

1. *Drug(s), concentration(s)*
2. *Instructions for administration*   if boluses
   - drug dose
   - interval between injections
   if infusion
   - loading dose
   - infusion rate
3. *Instructions for treating breakthrough pain*
4. *Maintain IV route and access to drugs for immediate use*
5. *A statement to eliminate the ordering of CNS depressants by others*
6. *Monitoring instructions*   for effects of opioids
   for effects of local anesthetics
   - bradycardia
   - hypotension
   - extensive sensory or motor block
7. *Observations that should be communicated to the anesthesiologist (e.g. systolic blood pressure less than . . . mmHg)*
8. *Instructions for the treatment of side effects*   respiratory depression
   nausea and/or vomiting
   pruritus
   urinary retention
9. *Instructions about concurrent use of other CNS depressants*
10. *Instruction about whom to contact if problems occur*
11. *Date, time, signature*

Box 6.6
Reproduced from Ready et al (1995) with permission

NURSING PROCEDURE PROTOCOLS

The format of nursing procedure protocols for epidural and intrathecal analgesia will vary with each institution, but there are elements that need to be included in each, regardless of format. These are listed in **Box 6.7**.

Elements of epidural and intrathecal nursing policies and protocols

1. A statement of the institution policy towards accreditation for nursing staff responsible for a patient with epidural or intrathecal analgesia.
2. A statement indicating who has responsibility for writing epidural or intrathecal orders.
3. Mechanisms for the checking and discarding of opioids.
4. Guidelines for the suitability, or otherwise, of patients for epidural or intrathecal analgesia.
5. Guidelines for preoperative patient education (technique should be explained in detail by the anesthesiologist).
6. Monitoring and documentation requirements.
7. Availability and use of drugs to treat side effects.
8. Instructions for the administration of bolus doses (including the need to aspirate the catheter using a small syringe to check for presence of CSF or blood).
9. Instructions for checking the amount of drug delivered (from the infusion pump display) against the amount remaining in the syringe.
10. Detailed instruction on the setting up and programming of infusion pumps.
11. Instructions for checking the catheter insertion site, redressing of the site if needed and for the labelling of the epidural (or intrathecal) catheters.
12. Instruction for checking and documenting completeness of epidural catheter tip once removed.
13. Instructions for mobilization of the patient.
14. Management of equipment faults and alarms.
15. Instructions about whom to call if assistance or advice is required.

Box 6.7

DAILY MANAGEMENT

Standard orders are used for the initial prescription of epidural and intrathecal analgesia but these orders may not be effective for all patients. Daily evaluation (or more often if required) will allow assessment of the effectiveness of analgesia and the treatment of side effects, including the need for changes to the prescription or analgesic technique and an assessment of catheter-related complications; an overall assessment of the patient, including the possibility of nonanalgesia-related complications, and any concurrent medication orders; and discussion with the patient and the patient's nurse and doctor of the assessment and treatment plans.

Advantage should be taken of the opportunity to encourage patients and staff to use the pain relief provided by epidural and intrathecal analgesia to exercise and mobilize (including showering) – better analgesia alone will not necessarily improve patient outcome. Patients receiving epidural infusions of a mixture of local anesthetic and opioid drugs can sit out of bed or walk about, but this should be done slowly and with two assistants because of the risk of leg weakness, loss of position sense or postural hypotension.

Guidelines for daily evaluation of epidural analgesia suggested by the American Society of Anesthesiologists are listed in **Box 6.8**.

Elements of epidural analgesia daily care

The following items should be included during a bedside evaluation at least once a day while epidural analgesia is administered.

1. **Note** the dose of analgesic medication given in the past 24 hours, and present parameters of bolus administration or infusion pump settings (if used).
2. **Evaluate** pain intensity both at rest and with operation-specific convalescent activity (e.g. passive continuous movement for knee replacement or chest physical therapy for thoracotomy). If pain is out of proportion to the surgical procedure, the number of days elapsed postoperatively and analgesic therapy given, consider whether another cause is present (e.g. surgical complication, personality disorder, opioid tolerance) and initiate appropriate evaluation, including communication with the surgeon and/or other consultant physicians.

3. **Determine** whether side effects are present. Assess each side effect in the context of the type of operation and days elapsed since the operation. Decide whether the side effect is in proportion to the operation, the number of days postoperatively, and the amount of opioid and other medications given. For sedation, as an example, note other concurrent drug therapy, as well as the patient's physical status, and decide whether to undertake other tests (e.g. analysis of glucose, electrolytes, arterial blood gas, calcium, magnesium, electrocardiogram).

4. **Perform** a problem-oriented physical examination (e.g. surgical site, presence of rales, venous thrombosis, sensory/motor function). Included in the physical examination should be an examination of the catheter site and brief neurological evaluation for evidence of catheter-related complications (e.g. change in position, infection, hematoma), as well as an evaluation for cardiovascular stability (especially in patients receiving local anesthetics). Note the current vital signs (heart rate, respiratory rate, blood pressure) and compare them with the last evaluation. If these are unstable or unsatisfactory, consider suitable diagnostic investigations (e.g. hematocrit, electrocardiogram).

5. **Adjust** drug doses, administration interval, infusion pump settings, or change to a different analgesic, as appropriate.

6. **Note** concurrent medications and decide whether the patient would benefit from changing the overall regimen (e.g. simplifying to avert drug interactions), or employing adjuvant medications or nonpharmacological therapies, and if so, order these.

7. **Evaluate** overall patient satisfaction with current care.

8. **Evaluate** patient's response(s) to prior adjustments of pain therapy or addition of adjuvants (e.g. for nausea or anxiety). Make changes in pain and adjuvant therapy as indicated.

9. **Evaluate** patient's suitability for making the transition to simpler alternatives (e.g. oral analgesics).

10. **Discuss** the assessment and plan with the patient and the patient's nurse and/or surgeon when appropriate.

11. **Document** findings, impression and plan in the hospital chart.

12. **Ensure** availability of personnel with appropriate expertise to deal with questions or problems at any time.

Box 6.8
Reproduced from Ready et al (1995) with permission

SUBSEQUENT ANALGESIC REGIMENS

Unlike patient-controlled analgesia (PCA), epidural and intrathecal analgesic doses cannot be used as a guide for the prescription of subsequent opioid regimens. If PCA or other parenteral or oral opioids are used following intrathecal analgesia, smaller than normal doses are suggested until the risk of delayed respiratory depression is past and until the response of the patient to these doses is seen (e.g. half the normal PCA bolus dose).

There should be some overlap of pain therapies so that the subsequent regimen has time to have an effect before the first is withdrawn. If there is to be a change in clinical responsibility for the pain management of the patient, then this change needs to be clearly understood by all staff.

COMPLICATIONS

Complications of epidural and intrathecal analgesia may be related to the *equipment* (needle, catheter or infusion pumps), *inadequate analgesia* or the *side effects of the drugs*.

PROBLEMS RELATED TO THE EQUIPMENT

Complications related to insertion of an epidural or spinal needle or catheter

Management of complications related to the insertion of an epidural or spinal needle or catherer is summarized in **Box 6.9**.

Nerve and spinal cord injury   Injuries to nerves or the spinal cord are very rare complications. In some instances, neurological problems have occurred in the presence of, but not because of, these forms of analgesia. For example, paraplegia can result from other causes of decreased spinal cord blood flow such as hypotension (from causes other than the epidural or spinal blockade), increased abdominal venous pressure leading to increased epidural venous pressure, injury to an anterior spinal artery or cross-clamping of an aorta; and damage to lumbosacral nerve

> ### Management of complications related to insertion of epidural or spinal needles or catheters
>
> | | |
> |---|---|
> | *Nerve or spinal cord injury* | Immediate neurological assessment |
> | *Dural puncture headache* | Bed rest |
> | | Analgesia (simple or opioid) |
> | | Hydrate (oral or IV) |
> | | Blood patch |
> | *Epidural hematoma* | Immediate neurosurgical assessment |
> | (early signs and symptoms include | CT/MRI scan |
> | back pain or nerve root pain, back | Urgent surgical decompression if |
> | tenderness) | neurological changes develop due |
> | | to nerve or spinal cord |
> | | compression |
> | *Epidural abscess* | Antibiotics |
> | (early signs and symptoms as for | Immediate neurosurgical assessment |
> | epidural hematoma, with or without | CT/MRI scan |
> | fever) | Urgent surgical decompression if |
> | | neurological changes develop due |
> | | to nerve or spinal cord |
> | | compression |
> | *Epidural catheter migration* | Treat as for complications of |
> | (opioid and/or local anesthetic | excessive opioid or local |
> | intended for epidural analgesia may | anesthetic doses |
> | be delivered into the CSF or | |
> | epidural blood vessel) | |

Box 6.9

roots may occur during labor and delivery due to pressure of the presenting fetal part. Any signs and symptoms of spinal cord or nerve root injury require immediate neurological assessment.

Small gauge microspinal catheters (28 and 32 gauge) have been used for continuous spinal anesthesia but their continued use into the postoperative period was not common. Reports of nerve injury (particularly cauda equina syndrome, characterized by alterations in sphincter function and perineal sensory loss) following the use of these catheters to administer hyperbaric lidocaine (lignocaine) (see Chapter 3) have led to their withdrawal from use in many countries.

Headache after dural puncture Whenever the dura mater is punctured, intentionally or unintentionally, leakage of CSF can occur. This can, in turn, lead to a decrease in CSF pressure and tension on meningeal vessels and nerves which can result in a 'dural puncture' headache. The incidence of headache following dural puncture is less with smaller needles, certain types of needle and in older patients.

The signs and symptoms are fairly typical and usually occur 1–2 days after the puncture. The headache is usually bifrontal and/or occipital, worse if the patient sits or strains, and may be associated with nausea and vomiting, photophobia, depression and ringing in the ears. Severe cases may also be associated with diplopia or other cranial nerve palsy from traction on these nerves. Very rarely, intracranial bleeding has resulted.

Initial treatment consists of bed rest, hydration and analgesia (simple or opioid). In some centers caffeine has been used with success. If these measures are not effective a 'blood patch' can be performed. This means that another epidural needle is inserted and, in a sterile manner, 10 ml of the patient's blood is injected into the epidural space. This effectively seals the hole through which the CSF is leaking and relief from the headache is almost immediate in 95% of cases. Blood patches may occasionally cause minor backache or headache.

Epidural hematoma Epidural hematomas are very rare but can follow trauma to an epidural blood vessel with epidural or spinal needles or catheters. They have also been reported to occur spontaneously in patients with bleeding disorders or in those taking anticoagulant medications.

The first signs and symptoms are often vague. The patient may complain of increasing back pain, root pain or back tenderness. The epidural or spinal anesthetic block may be patchy or may last for longer than the expected postoperative time. Neurological changes (sensory and/or motor) may develop as the hematoma increases in size and compresses nerve roots or spinal cord. An immediate neurosurgical consultation and computerized tomographic (CT) or magnetic resonance imaging (MRI) scans should be requested. Urgent surgical decompression within 12 hours gives the best chance of full recovery.

Infection   Meningitis or epidural space infections or abscesses are also rare complications of epidural and intrathecal analgesia. The infection may result from direct needle or catheter inoculation, infusion of contaminated fluid, tracking along the catheter from a superficial infection at the site of insertion, or from hematogenous spread during episodes of bacteremia. As with epidural hematomas, infections can also occur spontaneously.

The early signs and symptoms of an epidural abscess can be indistinct. The patient may complain of increasing back pain, root pain or back tenderness. The patient may or may not be febrile. Epidural space infections may be treated conservatively, in the first instance, with antibiotics. However, the development of any neurological changes due to nerve root or spinal cord compression indicates the need for urgent surgical treatment. An immediate neurosurgical consultation and CT or MRI scans should be requested. As with an epidural hematoma, urgent surgical decompression within 12 hours gives the best chance of full recovery.

Should infection occur, early recognition and treatment will reduce the risk of more serious sequelae. The epidural catheter insertion site should therefore be inspected daily and note taken of the patient's temperature. The catheter should be removed if there is any sign of inflammation or infection and the tip of the catheter sent for culture. Any significant infection should be treated with the appropriate antibiotics. If the patient's fever is greater than would be expected in the immediate postoperative period, consideration should be given to removal of the catheter.

The development of signs and symptoms of an epidural abscess may be delayed, even until well after the patient has been discharged from hospital. Patients must be aware that they should report to the hospital immediately if any problems are noted.

Catheter migration   Very rarely a catheter placed in the epidural space will migrate into the intrathecal space or an epidural blood vessel. If intrathecal migration is not recognized, large doses of drugs (opioids and/or local anesthetics) intended for epidural administration will be delivered into the CSF. Complications due to catheter migration will be more obvious and of greater magnitude if bolus doses of epidural opioid and/or local anesthetic drugs are given.

Epidural catheter or filter problems

Disconnection of the catheter from the epidural filter can result in contamination of the end of the catheter and migration of bacteria in the epidural infusion solution. If this disconnection is seen and it is important for epidural analgesia to continue, it may be reasonable to reconnect the catheter after the outside of it has been wiped with an antiseptic solution and a couple of centimeters trimmed from its end with sterile scissors. This should not be done without consulting the anesthesiologist responsible for the epidural analgesia.

Kinking of the catheter can occur, making infusion or administration of a bolus dose difficult or impossible. The length of the catheter should be checked for obvious kinks; if none is visible it might be worth pulling the catheter back by a centimeter. Slight flexion of the patient's back may also overcome the problem.

Leaking filters should be replaced as, again, there is a risk of contamination of the epidural solution. If the catheter appears to be leaking at the insertion site it may be that the tip of the catheter is no longer in the epidural space but lying in subcutaneous tissue (a small fluid collection under the dressing at the site of catheter insertion is not unusual). In this case, analgesia is likely to be inadequate.

The catheter should be inspected on removal to ensure that the tip is complete. If it is not (the tip may be sheared off, for example, if it is withdrawn through the inserting needle), the patient should be told and details entered in the patient's record. However, the catheter material is inert and surgical removal of the tip is usually unnecessary.

Infusion pumps

Operator error can lead to misprogramming of infusion pumps; infusion pumps may malfunction; or patients may attempt to interfere with the running of the pumps (unlike PCA machines, drugs contained in most infusion or syringe pumps are easily accessible to all).

INADEQUATE ANALGESIA

Epidural analgesia

An assessment of the patient must first exclude other causes of pain, e.g. a postsurgical complication. The catheter site should be checked and a bolus dose of the opioid or opioid/local anesthetic solution given (not all hospitals allow nursing staff to do this). The rate of any infusion can also be increased. If analgesia remains inadequate, correct placement of the catheter should be verified using a 'test dose' of 3–8 ml of local anesthetic solution, e.g. 0.25% bupivacaine or 1% lidocaine (lignocaine). This 'test dose' should be given by an anesthesiologist. A bilateral sensory block means that the catheter is in the epidural space and larger doses (increased concentration or increased volume) of analgesic drug are needed. If the resulting sensory block is unilateral, the catheter tip may have left the epidural space through an intervertebral foramen. The catheter should be withdrawn 1–2 cm and another 'test dose' given. Lack of any sensory block indicates that the epidural catheter is no longer in the epidural space and the catheter will need to be reinserted or an alternative method of analgesia prescribed.

Intrathecal analgesia

Usually intrathecal opioids are administered as a single dose so that if analgesia is inadequate, supplementation with oral or parenteral opioids will be required. As these may increase the risk of respiratory depression, smaller than average doses (e.g. half the normal bolus dose for PCA) should be administered initially and increased only if they prove to be inadequate.

SIDE EFFECTS RELATED TO THE DRUGS

Possible side effects of epidural and intrathecal opioids and local anesthetics are outlined earlier in this chapter (see **Box 6.3**). Side effects will be exaggerated if doses intended for epidural administration are inadvertently given directly into the CSF.

Management of inadequate analgesia and side effects of epidural and intrathecal analgesia

Inadequate analgesia

Epidural analgesia

Give a bolus dose of opioid or opioid/local anesthetic solution and increase the rate of an infusion

Check position of catheter using a 'test dose' of 3–8 ml of local anesthetic (e.g. 1% lidocaine or 0.25% bupivacaine) and test for level of sensory block with cold or alcohol (test dose to be administered by an anesthesiologist only)

A bilateral block indicates need for increased dose (increased infusion rate or concentration of local anesthetic)

If block is unilateral withdraw catheter and give another test dose

If test dose shows no block the catheter is displaced. Order alternative analgesia or reinsert catheter

Intrathecal analgesia

Carefully administer alternative analgesia

Side effects

Nausea/vomiting

Administer antiemetics (change if ineffective)

Decrease the size of the bolus dose or the rate of the epidural infusion

Consider other possible causes

Change to another opioid

Lie patient flat and minimize movement until treatment has had time to work

Pruritus

Change to another opioid

Administer small doses of IV naloxone or an opioid agonist-antagonist

? Administer an antihistamine (watch for sedation)

Sedation/respiratory depression	Sedation score 2, respiratory rate > 8/min: reduce the size of bolus doses and/or the rate of infusion
	Sedation score 2, respiratory rate < 8/min: reduce the bolus dose and/or infusion rate, consider naloxone
	Sedation score 3 (regardless of respiratory rate): administer naloxone and stop the infusion
	A decrease in opioid concentration may be required
Urinary retention	Try small doses of IV naloxone
	Catheterize – 'in-out' or indwelling
Hypotension	Look for causes of hypovolemia
	Administer IV fluids +/− vasopressors
	Stop/reduce (often only temporarily) infusion
Numbness/weakness	Check for catheter migration (into CSF)
(opioid + local anesthetic combination)	Stop infusion for a short while, restart at a lower rate
	Consider reducing local anesthetic concentration

Box 6.10

Management of inadequate analgesia and side effects of epidural and intrathecal analgesia is summarized in **Box 6.10**.

PATIENT-CONTROLLED EPIDURAL ANALGESIA

Although epidural analgesia has been shown to provide superior pain relief, patient satisfaction is often higher with intravenous patient-controlled analgesia (IV-PCA). Patient-controlled epidural analgesia (PCEA) combines the benefits of better analgesia with the advantages of patient control. Experience with PCEA for the management of acute pain outside obstetric units is still somewhat limited, but both opioids and combinations of opioid and local anesthetic drugs have been used.

As with IV-PCA, a loading dose should be given before PCEA is commenced. Unlike IV-PCA, a continuous (background) infusion is frequently ordered – whether this infusion is necessary remains to be seen. Although there needs to be more investigation into ideal doses and lock-out intervals for each of the drugs, the parameters that have been used by some groups are listed in **Box 6.11**.

Patient-controlled epidural analgesia			
Drug	Bolus dose	Lock-out interval (min)	Background infusion
Morphine	0.2 mg	10	+/− 0.4 mg/hr
Meperidine (pethidine)	20–30 mg	15–30	
Fentanyl	0.015–0.02 mg	5	
Hydromorphone	0.15–0.3 mg	15	
0.125% Bupivacaine + 1–5 µg/ml fentanyl	3–4 ml	10	+/−3–6 ml/hr

Box 6.11

REFERENCES AND FURTHER READING

Ballantyne J.C., Loach A.B. and Carr D.B. (1988) Itching after epidural and spinal opiates. *Pain* **33**, 149–160.

Benedetti C. (1987) Intraspinal analgesia: an historical overview. *Acta Anaesthesiologica Scandinavica* **31**, suppl. 85, 17–24.

Chung J.H. and Harris S.N. (1992) Common side effects associated with spinal opioids and their treatment. In *Acute Pain – Mechanisms and Management* (eds Sinatra R.S., Hord A.H., Ginsberg B. and Preble L.M.). Mosby Year Book, St Louis.

Cooper D.W. and Turner G. (1993) Patient-controlled extradural analgesia to compare bupivacaine, fentanyl and bupivacaine with fentanyl in the treatment of postoperative pain. *British Journal of Anaesthesia* **70**, 503–507.

Cousins M.J. and Mather L.E. (1984) Intrathecal and epidural administration of opioids. *Anesthesiology* **61**, 276–310.

Plummer J.L., Cmielewski G.D., Reynolds G.K., Gourlay G.K. and Cherry D.A. (1990) Influence of polarity on dose response relationships of intrathecal opioids in rats. *Pain* **40**, 339–347.

Ready L.B., Chadwick H.S. and Ross B. (1987) Age predicts effective epidural morphine dose after abdominal hysterectomy. *Anesthesia and Analgesia* **66**, 1215–1218.

Ready L.B., Loper K.A., Nessly M. and Wild L. (1991) Postoperative epidural morphine is safe on surgical wards. *Anesthesiology* **75**, 452–456

Ready L.B., Ashburn M., Caplan R.A., Carr D.B., Connis R.T., Dixon C.L., Hubbard L. and Rice L.J. (1995) Practice Guidelines for Acute Pain Management in the Perioperative Setting – a report of the American Society of Anesthesiologists Task Force on Pain Management, Acute Pain Section. *Anesthesiology* **82**: 1071–1081.

Sinatra R.S. (1992) Spinal opioid analgesia: an overview. In *Acute Pain – Mechanisms and Management* (eds Sinatra R.S., Hord A.H., Ginsberg B. and Preble L.M.). Mosby Year Book, St Louis.

VadeBoncouer T.R. and Ferrante F.M. (1993) Epidural and subarachnoid opioids. In *Postoperative Pain Management* (eds Ferrante F.M. and VadeBoncouer T.R.). Churchill Livingstone, New York.

Wang J.K., Nauss L.A. and Thomas J.E. (1979) Pain relief by intrathecally applied morphine in man. *Anesthesiology* **50**, 149–151.

Wildsmith J.A. and McLure J.H. (1991) Anticoagulant drugs and central nerve blockade. *Anaesthesia* **46**, 613–614.

Yaksh T.L. and Rudy T.A. (1976) Analgesia mediated by a direct spinal action of narcotics. *Science* **192**, 1357–1358.

APPENDIX

Examples of standard orders for epidural analgesia, reproduced with permission of the Acute Pain Services at the Royal Adelaide Hospital, Adelaide, Australia and the University of Washington Medical Center., Seattle, Wash., USA.

6A Royal Adelaide Hospital Acute Pain Service epidural/intrathecal opioid ar algesia standard orders.

6B University of Washington Acute Pain Service epidural analgesia physician orders.

ROYAL ADELAIDE HOSPITAL

UR 72.1

ACUTE PAIN SERVICE
EPIDURAL/INTRATHECAL
OPIOID ANALGESIA
Standard Orders

Unit Record No.: _____

Surname: _____

Given Names: _____

Date of Birth: _____ Sex: _____

1. No systemic opioids or sedatives to be given except as ordered by the APS.

2. Naloxone 400 micrograms at bedside.

3. Oxygen at .... 1/min via nasal specs or .... mask.

4. Maintain IV access for 24 hours after the last dose of epidural/intrathecal opioid.

5. **Monitoring and documentation:**

   a) Record pain score, sedation score and respiratory rate hourly for 12 hours and then 2 hourly.

      Omit pain score if asleep.

   In addition:

   b) If bolus doses are used, stay with the patient for 5 mins watching for respiratory depression or sedation and 20 mins after injection record pain score, sedation score and respiratory rate.

   c) If an epidural infusion is used, record total dose or volume infused at each monitoring interval.

   d) If local anaesthetics or "cocktail" are used, also record:

      *blood pressure and heart rate every 5 mins for 20 mins after each bolus dose.

      *blood pressure and heart rate at each monitoring interval.

6. For inadequate analgesia or other problems related to the epidural, page the rostered APS anaesthetist.

   After 1730 hours this will be the 2nd on-call ESS anaesthetic registrar.

7. **OPIOID ORDER:** *(for epidural PCA, epidural opioid/LA mixtures or intrathecal opioids, place appropriate label below)*

148

APS EPIDURAL/INTRATHECAL OPIOIDS

a) Drug .... Concentration ....mg/ml

b) Bolus dose .... to .... mg (................. to .... ml) 2 hourly prn

   Bolus dose .... to .... mg (................. to .... ml) 2 hourly prn
   (Initial. date and time any change to the orders)

c) Infusion rate .... to .... mg (................. to .... ml) per hour

d) Initial dose .... mg (................. ml) given by Dr .... Time ....

   Epidural catheter inserted by Dr ....

e) If sedation score = 2, reduce bolus dose and/or infusion rate.

8. **TREATMENT OF SIDE EFFECTS:**

   a) **Respiratory depression.**
      If sedation score = 3 OR respiratory rate less than 8/min AND sedation score = 2 or 3,
      give 400 micrograms NALOXONE IV stat. Repeat PRN. Cease epidural infusion. Call the APS.

   b) **Nausea/vomiting.**
      Give METOCLOPRAMIDE 10mg IV 4 HOURLY PRN. If metoclopramide ineffective, give
      DROPERIDOL 250 micrograms IV 6 hourly PRN (dilute as in APS procedure book).

   c) **Severe itching or urinary retention.**
      Give 100 micrograms naloxone IV. Repeat every 10 mins PRN up to a total of 400 micrograms.

9. **SIGNATURE OF ANAESTHETIST** .... DATE ....
   (Print ....) TIME ....

10. Cease above orders, remove epidural catheter. Signature .... Date/time ....

11. Catheter removed and complete. Signature of RN .... Date/time ....

APPENDIX 6B

☐ EPIDURAL OPIOID	☐ EPIDURAL OPIOID / LOCAL ANESTHETIC MIXTURE
OPERATING ROOM DOSE: Drug _____ Mg _____ Time _____ **DRUG FOR CONTINUING EPIDURAL ANALGESIA:** ☐ PF MORPHINE (1mg/ml) _____ mg q 6–12 h. ☐ FENTANYL (10 mcg/ml normal saline) 　Infuse _____ mcg (_____ ml) per h. ☐ MEPERIDINE (2 mg/ml normal saline) 　Infuse _____ mg (_____ ml) per h. ☐ OTHER: Drug _____ Conc _____ 　Dose _____ Interval _____	**INFUSION BEGUN at** _____ **hours.** **MIXTURE:** ☐ BUPIVACAINE 1/16% (O.625 mg/ml normal saline) ☐ BUPIVACAINE 1/8% (1.25 mg/ml normal saline) **PLUS** ☐ FENTANYL (4 mcg/ml normal saline) **or** ☐ PF MORPHINE (0.1 mg/ml normal saline) **or** ☐ MEPERIDINE (2 mg/ml normal saline) **or** ☐ OTHER: Opioid _____ Conc _____ **INFUSE at** _____ **ml per h.**
BREAKTHROUGH PAIN: FENTANYL 50 mcg (1.0 ml) into epidural catheter q 3 h prn.	**BREAKTHROUGH PAIN:** FENTANYL 50 mcg (1.0 ml) into epidural catheter q 3 h prn.
MONITORING: Respiratory rate and sedation scale q 1 h for first 24 hours; then q 4 h.	**MONITORING:** A. BP/Pulse from start of infusion q 30 min x 3 h; then q 1 h x 24 h; then q 4 h. B. Resp rate & sedation scale q 1 h for first 24 h; then 4 h. C. Sensory level q 8 h. D. Motor function q 4 h. E. Postural BP/P prior to first ambulation.
NOTIFY APS FOR THE FOLLOWING: A. RR < 8/min. B. Sedation scale = 3. C. pCO2 > 50 mm Hg. D. Inadequate analgesia or other problems related to epidural.	**NOTIFY APS FOR THE FOLLOWING:** A. BP < _____ mm Hg and/or P < _____ /min. B. RR < 8/min. C. Sedation scale = 3. D. pCO2 > 50 mm Hg. E. Numbness above nipples and/or inability to bend knees. F. Postural BP drop > 15 mm Hg and/or HR increase > 20/min. G. Inadequate analgesia or other problems related to epidural.

KEEP AT BEDSIDE:
NALOXONE 0.4 mg

KEEP AT BEDSIDE:
NALOXONE 0.4 mg
EPHEDRINE 25 mg/5 ml (i.e. 5 mg/ml)

1. Maintain IV access (drip or peripheral lock with flushes) until epidural analgesia discontinued.
2. **No narcotics or other CNS depressants** to be given except as ordered by Acute Pain Service.
3. **Epidural Analgesia not to be discontinued** except by the Acute Pain Service.
4. **PRN Treatments:**
   A. NALOXONE 0.4 mg **IV stat** for sedation scale = **3 plus** RR < 8 per minute. Call Acute Pain Service.
   B. METOCLOPRAMIDE 10 mg IV q 4 h prn for nausea/vomiting. **In addition, if age < 60 years**, TRANSDERMAL SCOPOLAMINE PATCH to either mastoid area. Change q 72 h prn.
   C. DIPHENHYDRAMINE 25 mg, IV or PO q 6 h prn for severe itching.
   D. For urinary retention, "in and out" bladder catheter prn.
   E. If age < 60 years, TRIAZOLAM 0.125 mg PO qhs prn. MR x 1.

Dr. _____ on the Acute Pain Service was notified about this patient at _____ hours.

DATE	TIME	PHYSICIAN SIGNATURE

UNIVERSITY OF WASHINGTON MEDICAL CENTERS
HARBORVIEW MEDICAL CENTER
UNIVERSITY OF WASHINGTON MEDICAL CENTER
SEATTLE, WASHINGTON

ACUTE PAIN SERVICE EPIDURAL ANALGESIA PHYSICIAN ORDERS

UH 0949 REV NOV 92

WHITE - MEDICAL RECORD
CANARY - PHARMACY
PINK - NURSING

PT. NO.

NAME

D.O.B.

151

CHAPTER 7

OTHER DRUGS USED IN ACUTE PAIN MANAGEMENT

Nonsteroidal anti-inflammatory drugs;

Nitrous oxide;

Alpha-2-adrenergic agents;

Tricyclic antidepressants;

Anticonvulsant drugs;

Anxiolytic drugs

Drugs other than opioids and local anesthetics may also be used in the treatment of acute pain, either as the sole agent or as adjuvant medication.

NONSTEROIDAL ANTI-INFLAMMATORY DRUGS

The analgesic and anti-inflammatory properties of the bark of willow and other plants have been known for centuries. The active ingredient in willow bark is *salicin*, which can be converted to salicylic acid. The compounds obtained from natural sources were expensive and were soon replaced by synthetic salicylates.

Most nonsteroidal anti-inflammatory drugs (NSAIDs) exhibit a spectrum of analgesic, anti-inflammatory and antipyretic actions. There is a 'ceiling' effect to the analgesia produced by these drugs, when further increases in dose do not result in additional pain relief. There appears to be little if any difference in analgesic efficacy between the different NSAIDs, although differences may exist in their anti-inflammatory activity and the incidence of side effects. Most are given orally or rectally, although some

– e.g. ketorolac, tenoxicam and diclofenac – can be given by injection.

The NSAIDs may be used as the sole method of pain relief (for mild to moderate pain), or in combination with other analgesic drugs such as opioids. When used in combination with opioids, they have resulted in a 20–40% reduction in opioid requirements. This 'opioid sparing' is, however, only worth while if it results in better analgesia or a decrease in opioid-related side effects. As yet, there is no consistent evidence to show that 'opioid sparing' does have this effect. When NSAIDs are used *instead* of opioids, a significant reduction in side effects is seen. Because NSAIDs can produce a variety of undesirable adverse effects, the potential risks of their use should always be weighed against the possible benefits.

The NSAIDs act by inhibiting the enzyme cyclo-oxygenase and therefore the synthesis of prostaglandins, prostacyclin and thromboxane A_2. It is thought that prostaglandins released during tissue damage sensitize nerve endings to the effects of mechanical or chemical stimuli by lowering the threshold of the pain receptors. There is also increasing evidence that a central mechanism of action augments the peripheral analgesic actions of NSAIDs.

Prostaglandins are found in most body tissues, with high concentrations occurring in the distal tubules of the kidney, the gastrointestinal mucosa, the liver and inflamed tissue. As a result, inhibition of prostaglandin synthesis can have a number of effects.

Nonsteroidal anti-inflammatory drugs are rapidly absorbed from the gastrointestinal tract. Most are metabolized in the liver and the metabolites excreted by the kidney. Clearance is reduced in the elderly and those with renal disease.

ADVERSE EFFECTS

Gastrointestinal

Erosions of the gastrointestinal tract (especially the stomach) can develop. They are due to local irritation of the mucosa as well as decreases in mucus production and mucosal blood flow and increased gastric acid secretion, mediated by reductions in prostaglandin levels. Thus, the problem may be lessened but not avoided altogether if the drugs are given by parenteral or rectal routes. The H_2-blocker drugs (e.g. cimetidine, ranitidine) may be effective in preventing NSAID-induced gastric erosions.

Gastric irritation, dyspepsia and ulceration (which may be silent until a bleed or perforation occurs) may develop at any time, but are less likely with short-term treatment. Pre-existing peptic ulcer disease may be exacerbated.

Renal
If effective circulating blood volume is decreased (e.g. as a result of hypovolemia or dehydration, hypotension, excessive use of diuretics, congestive cardiac failure or cirrhosis), vasodilatory renal prostaglandins are released to maintain renal blood flow and counteract the vasoconstrictive influences of catecholamines and angiotensin. A reduction in prostaglandin levels due to NSAID administration may result in decreases in renal blood flow and acute renal failure. Pre-existing renal impairment may increase this risk.

In the healthy patient renal blood flow is not normally prostaglandin-dependent. However, renal blood flow may be altered during anesthesia. Recently, six cases of acute renal failure have been reported (Adverse Drug Reactions Advisory Committee, 1994) following perioperative administration of ketorolac. These patients were relatively young (28–53 years), and, apart from administration of gentamicin in three of the cases, there were no identifiable predisposing factors.

Nonsteroidal anti-inflammatory drugs can cause sodium, potassium and water retention which may lead to edema in some patients. They may also reduce the effectiveness of antihypertensive therapy. Interstitial nephritis has also been reported.

Hematological
Aggregation of platelets depends on a balance between prostacyclin (from endothelial cells) and thromboxane A_2 (from platelets). The former is a vasodilator and inhibits platelet aggregation; the latter is a vasoconstrictor and stimulates platelet aggregation. Nonsteroidal anti-inflammatory drugs inhibit the synthesis of

both these factors and the net balance will determine the tendency to bleed.

Aspirin is particularly effective in inhibiting platelet function as it irreversibly inhibits platelet cyclo-oxygenase and effectively prolongs bleeding time for the life of the platelet (8–11 days). As platelets cannot regenerate the enzyme, recovery depends on the production of new platelets. Other NSAIDs reversibly inhibit platelet cyclo-oxygenase and the effect lasts only as long as the drugs remain in the blood (five half-lives). Increases in bleeding times have been reported with the use of NSAIDs.

Respiratory
Bronchospasm, related to cyclo-oxygenase inhibition, can occur in some asthmatic patients so NSAIDs should be used with caution in these people. Up to 20% of adult asthmatics may develop aspirin-induced asthma, and a cross-sensitivity does exist between aspirin and other NSAIDs. The triad of aspirin intolerance, nasal polyps and asthma is a definite contraindication to the use of these drugs.

Liver
Abnormalities in liver function tests may occur but are usually transient.

Other effects
Headache, anxiety, depression, confusion, dizziness and somnolence have all been reported, as have a variety of skin reactions and blood dyscrasias.

PRECAUTIONS AND CONTRAINDICATIONS
Before NSAIDs are prescribed, reference should be made to the appropriate product information sheet for each of these drugs, as precautions, contraindications, doses, permitted routes of administration and duration of therapy vary according to country and drug.

A newer and now commonly used NSAID is ketorolac. Its major advantage is its worldwide availability in an injectable (non-irritating) form. Reports of adverse events have led to continuing revisions of the product information sheet for ketorolac in many countries. **Box 7.1** summarizes some of the current precautions and contraindications listed in product information sheets (USA, UK and Australia) for ketorolac, these apply equally well to any NSAID used in the management of acute pain.

Possible precautions and contraindications to the use of ketorolac and other NSAIDs for acute pain management

- dehydration or hypovolemia from any cause
- pre-existing:
  renal impairment
  impaired hepatic function
  peptic ulcer disease (active or inactive)
  bleeding or coagulation disorders
  cerebrovascular bleeding
  cardiac failure
  gastrointestinal bleeding
- operations where there is a high risk of hemorrhage or where an absence of bleeding is important (e.g. eye surgery, neurosurgery and cosmetic surgery)
- aspirin-induced asthma or other severe asthma, especially if the triad of asthma, nasal polyps and sensitivity to aspirin is present
- hypersensitivity to aspirin or other NSAIDs
- concurrent use of:
  other NSAIDs
  diuretics
  other nephrotoxic medications, e.g. aminoglycosides
  anticoagulants
- children less than 16 years old
- pregnant and lactating women
- advanced age

Many perioperative factors may adversely affect renal blood flow and it may be wise to delay administration of NSAIDs until the postoperative period and until the patient is normovolemic and normotensive.

Box 7.1

DOSES

Suggested doses and duration of therapy vary according to each drug, each approved route of administration and each country. Reference should be made to the appropriate product information sheet.

ACETAMINOPHEN (PARACETAMOL)

Although an NSAID, acetaminophen (paracetamol) is only a weak inhibitor of peripheral prostaglandin synthesis. Its action is believed to result from inhibition of prostaglandin synthesis within the central nervous system. Acetaminophen is analgesic and antipyretic but only weakly anti-inflammatory.

Most of the drug is excreted by the kidney after glucuronide and sulfate conjugation in the liver. A small proportion is metabolized by the cytochrome P450 system to form the potentially hepato-toxic metabolite N-acetyl-*p*-benzoquinoneimine (NAPQI). This metabolite is normally inactivated by conjugation with hepatic glutathione to produce a nontoxic metabolite that is excreted in the urine. If large amounts of it are produced following large doses of acetaminophen, hepatic glutathione may be depleted and reaction of NAPQI with hepatic proteins increased. This may lead to hepatic necrosis. Susceptibility to hepatic toxicity is said to be increased in patients with chronic alcoholism. Reasons for this may include decreased hepatic levels of glutathione and/or higher levels of NAPQI.

Side effects of the drug are normally minimal.

Acetaminophen is usually given orally or rectally. However, an intravenous preparation of *propacetamol* has been released in some countries. This is a 'prodrug' which is rapidly hydrolysed in the body to acetaminophen.

NITROUS OXIDE

Nitrous oxide is commonly used in some countries as a combination of 50% nitrous oxide and 50% oxygen in premixed cylinders (Entonox). In other countries, the use of a mixing valve permits a variety of nitrous oxide and oxygen combinations to be used. A one-way demand valve allows delivery of the gas when the patient inspires, providing there is an airtight fit between face and mask or mouthpiece. The technique is inherently safe as it is self-administered and if the patient becomes too drowsy the mask will fall away from the face.

The onset of analgesia is rapid and some effect will be seen after four or five deep breaths. The offset of effect is also rapid so analgesia can only be maintained by repeated inhalations.

Duration of exposure should be limited because nitrous oxide can interfere with methionine synthetase activity, which in turn impairs DNA synthesis and folate metabolism resulting in bone marrow depression. For this reason nitrous oxide is usually only ordered for short, painful procedures, such as coughing and breathing exercises in patients with fractured ribs or removal of drains or dressings. It is normally used in combination with opioid or other analgesic therapies. In some institutions, concerns about environmental nitrous oxide levels limit the use of nitrous oxide in general wards.

CONTRAINDICATIONS

Nitrous oxide is contraindicated in the presence of air-containing spaces such as a pneumothorax or intracranial air. Gases equilibrate across permeable membranes so that concentrations on either side become equal. Nitrous oxide equilibrates rapidly; nitrogen much more slowly. If a patient breathes a mixture containing only oxygen and nitrous oxide, the concentration of nitrous oxide in any air containing space will rise rapidly. However, the concentration of nitrogen will fall much more slowly so that there is an overall increase in volume of the gas space. The use of nitrous oxide may rapidly increase (e.g. double) the size of any air-containing spaces. For the same reason, middle ear pressures can also rise.

α_2-ADRENERGIC AGENTS

The selective α_2 agonist, clonidine, has been used by oral, intravenous, epidural and intrathecal routes for the management of acute pain. Another α_2 agonist, dexmedetomidine (systemically administered), is used less frequently. The analgesic action of these drugs is centrally mediated, involving descending modulating pathways. Other effects of the drugs include:

- hypotension, bradycardia
- sedation, anxiolysis, dizziness
- dry mouth, decreased bowel motility
- diuresis

These effects limit the use of α_2 agonists as the sole analgesic agent. They are usually used in combination with opioids and result in reduced opioid requirements.

The exact role of these drugs has yet to be determined and their use in clinical practice is, as yet, uncommon. Clonidine has also been used in the treatment of opioid withdrawal (abstinence) syndrome. It is most effective in suppressing the autonomic symptoms of this syndrome.

TRICYCLIC ANTIDEPRESSANTS

Sleep disturbances and depression often accompany pain and have been associated with increased perceptions of pain intensity. Tricyclic antidepressants can help to normalize sleep cycles, often leading to a decrease in pain. They also have a centrally mediated analgesic action.

In cases where the duration of acute pain is more than a few days (e.g. after multiple injuries, repeated operations), these drugs can be very useful and may obviate the need for hypnotic drugs at night. Doses should start at the lower end of the recommended ranges, especially in the elderly. Doses can be increased after each couple of days if there are no side effects. Amitriptyline is commonly used, starting at a dose of 10–25 mg orally at night. Although antidepressant effects of these drugs may not be seen for 2–3 weeks after starting therapy, the effects on sleep pattern and pain may be seen within a couple of days.

The side effects of these drugs result mainly from their anticholinergic actions and include dry mouth, increased heart rate, blurred vision and urinary retention. Mild postural (orthostatic) hypotension and sedation can also occur, and narrow-angle glaucoma can be aggravated. More serious side effects are rare.

ANTICONVULSANT DRUGS

Anticonvulsant drugs, most commonly carbamazepine, stabilize excitable cell membranes and may be useful in the treatment of neuropathic pain (dysesthesias, burning or shooting pain). However, optimal effect may not be seen for weeks. Although most often used in the management of chronic pain, these drugs can be a useful adjunct to other acute pain therapies, e.g. for pain resulting from nerve damage after brachial plexus injury, fractured vertebra or fractured pelvis.

Carbamazepine is structurally related to the tricyclic antidepressants. It is often commenced at a dose of 100 mg orally every 12 hours, and increased after a few days if necessary and if there are no side effects. Blood levels should be checked and kept within the therapeutic range.

During long-term treatment, the most frequently reported side effects are blurred vision, drowsiness, ataxia and vertigo. Other adverse effects have included nausea and vomiting, transient leucopenia, aplastic anemia and hypersensitivity reactions.

ANXIOLYTIC DRUGS

Anxiety increases the perception of pain and analgesic use. In most instances, anxiety can be allayed by appropriate information and reassurance. In some cases anxiolytic drugs, such as benzodiazepines, will be required. Benzodiazepines may also help in the treatment of muscle spasm, for instance after spinal injury or surgery; they should be used with caution if administered concurrently with opioids, as they will increase the risk of respiratory depression. Small initial doses should be used and subsequent doses titrated to effect.

REFERENCES AND FURTHER READING

Adverse Drug Reactions Advisory Committee (1994) Ketorolac and renal failure. *Australian Adverse Drug Reactions Bulletin* **13**, 3.

Campbell W.B. (1992) Lipid derived autacoids: eicosanoids and platelet-activating factor. In *Goodman and Gilman's The Pharmacological Basis of Therapeutics* (eds Gilman A.J., Rall T.W., Nies A.J. and Taylor P.). McGraw-Hill International, Singapore.

Dahl J.B. and Kehlet H. (1991) Non-steroidal anti-inflammatory drugs: rationale for use in severe postoperative pain. *British Journal of Anaesthesia* **66**, 703–712.

Eisenach J.C. (1993) Overview: first international symposium on α_2-adrenergic mechanisms of spinal anesthesia. *Regional Anesthesia* **18**, 207–212.

Insel P. (1992) Analgesic-antipyretic and antiinflammatory agents: drugs employed in the treatment of rheumatoid arthritis and gout. In *Goodman and Gilman's The Pharmacological Basis of Therapeutics* (eds Gilman A.J., Rall T.W., Nies A.J. and Taylor P.). McGraw-Hill International, Singapore.

Kehlet H. and Mather L.E. (eds) (1992) The value of NSAIDs in the management of postoperative pain. *Drugs* **44**, Suppl. 5, 1–63.

Maze M. and Tranquilli W. (1991) Alpha–2 adrenoceptor agonists: defining the role in clinical anesthesia. *Anesthesiology* **74**, 581–605.

Power I. (1993) Aspirin-induced asthma. *British Journal of Anaesthesia* **71**, 619–621.

CHAPTER 8

OTHER TECHNIQUES USED IN ACUTE PAIN MANAGEMENT

◆

Nonpharmacologic management (cognitive-behavioral interventions/physical techniques);
Other local anesthetic techniques (interpleural analgesia; other nerve and plexus blocks; local infiltration)

There are a number of other techniques that can be used in the management of acute pain, either alone or in combination with other methods.

NONPHARMACOLOGIC MANAGEMENT

Nonpharmacologic methods can be either cognitive-behavioral or physical (**Box 8.1**). Alone, these strategies will usually not be effective for the treatment of most acute pain; if used, they should be to supplement the pharmacologic or invasive techniques described in earlier chapters.

COGNITIVE-BEHAVIORAL INTERVENTIONS

Intensity of acute pain is known to be influenced by a number of psychological, behavioral and social factors. Acute pain management should include an assessment and, if necessary, treatment of these factors as they can influence the patient's response to pain therapy.

Anxiety and fear commonly accompany acute pain and have been shown to increase the amount of pain perceived, analgesic requirements and the tendency to report normally nonpainful stimulation as pain. Depression has also been associated with higher pain ratings but is a less common response to acute pain.

> **Examples of nonpharmacologic interventions**
>
> | | |
> |---|---|
> | *Cognitive-behavioral* | Reassurance |
> | | Education/information |
> | | Relaxation |
> | | Imagery |
> | | Distraction |
> | | Biofeedback |
> | | Hypnosis |
> | *Physical* | Applications of heat and cold |
> | | Massage, exercise and immobilization |
> | | Transcutaneous nerve stimulation (TENS) |
>
> *Adapted from Carr et al (1992)*

Box 8.1

The meaning that a person attaches to pain can influence perception of pain intensity and ability to tolerate pain. For example, perceived pain may be different if an operation for cancer is curative compared with an operation that is palliative only.

Locus of control testing may show how patients will respond and adapt to surgical pain. Those with an 'internal' locus of control believe that they can, through their own behavior, exert control over their health. A perception of lack of control in this group increases anxiety. Those with an 'external' locus of control believe that what they do will have little or no influence on the outcome of their health and that their health is in the hands of fate, chance or other people. This latter group may be very dependent on the ward staff and may not manage well with techniques such as PCA. It is possible that up to 20% of patients find the responsibility for control stress-inducing.

Coping styles may also affect self-reports of pain and the ability to tolerate pain. Occasional discrepancies between pain behavior and a patient's self-report of pain may result from different coping skills, e.g. staff should not necessarily assume that a patient who is smiling, reading or sleeping is comfortable.

Cognitive-behavioral interventions aim to help patients understand more about their pain, alter their pain behavior and coping skills, change their perception of pain and take an active part in pain assessment and control. Education (see Chapter 9) and information about expected discomforts, ways to decrease pain and details of all procedures, can decrease anxiety, analgesic use and self-reports of pain.

Some reductions in pain, anxiety and analgesic requirements may also follow the use of simple relaxation strategies (e.g. controlled breathing, muscle relaxation), distraction techniques (e.g. music) and imagery (e.g. imagining pleasant events). These methods need not be complicated to be effective; they are easy to teach but need periodic reinforcement. Hypnosis and biofeedback require specialized training or equipment and are therefore not suitable for routine acute pain management.

PHYSICAL TECHNIQUES

Applications of heat or cold, massage, exercise and immobilization will help to relieve pain and muscle spasm. Widely used in the management of chronic pain, transcutaneous electrical nerve stimulation can also be used for the treatment of acute pain.

Transcutaneous electrical nerve stimulation

Transcutaneous electrical nerve stimulation (TENS) has been shown to be effective in reducing analgesic requirements and subjective reports of pain after some operations and other acute pain states. This technique may also be of benefit in alleviating the burning neuropathic pain that can follow nerve trauma, a pain that is often not very responsive to opioids. Normally, TENS is used in combination with other pain relief therapies and not as the sole means of treatment for acute pain.

The technique is simple, noninvasive, virtually free from side effects and allows patients some control over their own therapy. The battery-powered TENS unit generates a small electric current which is transmitted to electrodes placed on the skin. The best effect is achieved when the electrodes are placed over the nerve innervating the affected area, over the affected or adjacent dermatome, above and below the painful site or over trigger or acupuncture points. The amplitude and frequency of the current delivered to the nerves under the skin are varied by the patient according to the severity of the pain. The current is altered until it is low enough to produce only a comfortable buzzing or tingling on the skin.

There are two types of TENS stimulation: conventional, which works by the gate-control theory and is used most commonly; and acupuncture-like. Most of the experience with postoperative pain management has been gained with conventional TENS.

- *Conventional TENS* uses high-frequency currents which stimulate non-pain-producing large-diameter nerve fibres (Aβ). This 'closes the gate' in the dorsal horn and inhibits transmission of pain impulses along small-diameter, pain-producing nerve fibres (C and Aδ). Onset of the effect of conventional TENS is almost instantaneous.

- *Acupuncture-like TENS* uses lower frequency currents which are thought to stimulate the production and release of endorphins. This is a slow process and may take up to 60 minutes for an effect to be felt. The analgesia produced is reversible by naloxone.

Contraindications It is suggested that TENS be avoided during the first trimester of pregnancy and in patients with cardiac pacemakers. Electrical interference may disrupt normal cardiac pacemaker function – demand-type pacemakers may sense the stimulus from the TENS unit as cardiac activity.

Complications Skin irritation may occur at electrode sites but is rarely serious.

OTHER LOCAL ANESTHETIC TECHNIQUES

INTERPLEURAL ANALGESIA

Intercostal nerves can be blocked by injection of local anesthetic solution into the intercostal space just below each rib. The disadvantages of this block are that multiple injections may be needed, especially if the operation or injury is extensive. These need to be repeated whenever pain returns, as often as every 6–8 hours. Local anesthetic solution administered through intercostal catheters may spread over a number of intercostal spaces. However, an easier method of achieving multiple intercostal blocks at the same time without the need for repeated injections is to use an interpleural catheter.

Interpleural analgesia was first used for the management of acute pain in 1984. It has also gained popularity for the management of some chronic pain problems. The local anesthetic solution is injected into the interpleural space (between the parietal and visceral pleura) via an indwelling catheter (an epidural catheter is used). The local anesthetic drug spreads by capillary action around the lung and then diffuses back into the intercostal spaces, blocking multiple intercostal nerves. It also spreads to the thoracic sympathetic chain and splanchnic nerves and may reach the phrenic nerve, although no problems have been reported where normal doses have been used.

The local anesthetic agent most commonly used for interpleural analgesia is bupivacaine (0.25–0.5%). The addition of epinephrine (adrenaline) to the solution may decrease blood levels of the drug and lessen the risk of systemic toxicity. The local anesthetic drug can be given as repeated bolus doses or by infusion.

Indications

Interpleural analgesia is usually only used for unilateral pain, e.g. cholecystectomy, renal surgery, unilateral breast surgery and fractured ribs, although bilateral catheters have been inserted for more extensive operations or injuries. It has also been used for chronic pancreatitis, herpes zoster (where early use is said to reduce the incidence of postherpetic neuralgia) and in the treatment of reflex sympathetic dystrophy (RSD) of the upper limb.

The block works less well after thoracotomies but the incidence of successful blocks may be improved if the surgeon places the catheter in the paravertebral gutter and if the chest drain is clamped for 30 minutes after each bolus dose of local anesthetic drug.

Contraindications

Contraindications include disease states that may interfere with the spread of the local anesthetic; result in a more rapid uptake of the local anesthetic into the circulation; increase the risk or consequences of pneumothorax; or increase the risk of infection. Examples include:

- pleural inflammation, recent pneumonia
- pleural effusion, hemothorax, pneumothorax
- pleural fibrosis, adhesions
- bullous emphysema
- infection at the proposed site of insertion

Complications

Complications of the technique include:

- pneumothorax (including tension pneumothorax) – potentially more serious with nitrous oxide and positive pressure ventilation
- nerve or vessel trauma
- phrenic nerve block
- inadvertent injection into blood vessel or lung
- Horner's syndrome
- infection
- local anesthetic toxicity (see Chapter 3)

In many institutions the use of these blocks is confined to high-dependency or intensive care units, primarily because of the risk of local anesthetic toxicity.

Standard orders and nursing policies and procedures

Interpleural analgesia is normally initiated and managed by anesthesiologists. Standard orders and nursing policies and procedures are recommended for the management of this form of pain relief. Interpleural catheters should carry a clearly visible label.

Commonly used doses are: bolus doses of 20–30 ml 0.25–0.5% bupivacaine given as frequently as every 4–6 hours; or an infusion of 6–10 ml per hour of 0.25% bupivacaine. Epinephrine can be added to the solutions. Supplemental analgesia (e.g. opioids) may be required in some cases.

OTHER NERVE AND PLEXUS BLOCKS

Long-acting local anesthetic drugs used for nerve or plexus anesthesia (e.g. brachial plexus, sciatic and femoral nerves) can produce analgesia for up to 24 hours after a single injection. Infusions of local anesthetic solutions through indwelling catheters have been used for longer periods of continuous regional analgesia and sympathetic blockade.

Anesthesiologists will usually be responsible for the performance of these blocks and their continued management if an infusion is used. However, a femoral nerve block is easy to accomplish. It can provide rapid and excellent analgesia following a fractured femur as it reduces the spasm of the quadriceps muscle that inevitably accompanies this fracture and exacerbates the pain.

Femoral nerve block

The femoral nerve is blocked just below the inguinal ligament as the nerve enters the thigh lateral to the femoral artery. The needle (short-bevelled) should be inserted 2 cm below the inguinal ligament and 1 cm (or one finger's breadth) lateral to the artery and to a depth just below that of the artery. Paresthesias indicate that the needle has touched the nerve but it is not necessary to search for them with this particular block. If paresthesias have not been obtained, the local anesthetic solution should be injected in a fan-like fashion starting just lateral to the femoral artery and proceeding laterally.

Prior to the injection of 10–20 ml of local anesthetic solution (0.25–0.5% bupivacaine), negative aspiration of blood through the needle should be demonstrated. This should be repeated after every 5 ml to ensure that the needle has not entered a blood vessel. The injection should cease immediately if there is resistance or pain on injection as either can indicate injection of local anesthetic directly into nerve tissue. No block should be performed without intravenous access and the availability of resuscitation equipment and staff able to manage any of the complications that may arise from local anesthetic administration.

LOCAL INFILTRATION

Single injections of local anesthetic drugs into wounds can produce effective analgesia following minor operations, e.g. repair of inguinal hernia. Wound infiltration following more major operations has also been shown to be effective, but unless a catheter is placed in the wound, it only delays the time until other methods of analgesia are required.

REFERENCES AND FURTHER READING

Brown R.E. (1992) Transcutaneous electrical nerve stimulation for acute and postoperative pain. In *Acute Pain – Mechanisms and Management* (eds Sinatra R.S., Hord A.H., Ginsberg B. and Preble L.M.). Mosby Year Book, St Louis.

Carr D.B., Jacox A.K., Chapman C.R. et al. (1992) *Acute Pain Management: Operative or Medical Procedures and Trauma, Clinical Practice Guideline.* AHCPR Pub. No. 92–0032. Rockville, MD: Agency for Health Care Policy and Research, Public Health Service, US Department of Health and Human Services.

Melzack R. (1988) Psychological aspects of pain: implications for neural blockade. In *Neural Blockade in Clinical Anesthesia and Management of Pain* (eds Cousins M.J. and Bridenbaugh P.O.). J.B. Lippincott, Philadelphia.

Murphy D.F. (1993) Interpleural analgesia. *British Journal of Anaesthesia* **71**, 426–434.

Peck C.L. (1986) Psychological factors in acute pain management. In *Acute Pain Management* (eds M.J. Cousins and G.D. Phillips). Churchill Livingstone, New York.

VadeBoncouer T.R. (1993) Interpleural regional anesthesia. In *Postoperative Pain Management* (eds Ferrante F.M. and VadeBoncouer T.R.). Churchill Livingstone, New York.

VanDalfsen P.J. and Syrjala K.L. (1989) Psychological strategies in acute pain management. *Anesthesiology Clinics of North America* **7**, 171–181.

CHAPTER 9

EDUCATION

Nursing staff;

Medical staff;

Patients

One of the well-recognized reasons for past deficiencies in the management of acute pain has been inadequate education of nursing staff, medical staff and patients. Better education of all groups is necessary if the more sophisticated methods of pain relief (such as patient-controlled and epidural analgesia) are to be managed safely and effectively and if better results are to be gained from more conventional methods of pain relief (such as intermittent opioid injections).

MEDICAL STAFF

Education of junior medical staff needs to include all aspects of the management of acute pain. While they will not be directly responsible for the more advanced, newer methods of pain relief, they must have a sound working knowledge of them so that they are aware of possible complications and drug interactions, and can explain the techniques to both the patients and their relatives. Responsibility for the more conventional methods of analgesia is often delegated to junior medical staff, and a better understanding of the drugs and techniques available can help to improve the effectiveness of these forms of pain relief.

Current teaching usually includes extensive information about the anatomy, physiology and theory of pain, but lacks sufficient practical detail.

NURSING STAFF

Ward nursing staff play a key role in ensuring that all forms of analgesia, simple or sophisticated, are safely and effectively managed. Therefore a nursing education program is essential.

NURSING EDUCATION PROGRAM

The education requirements are twofold – general and specialized.

General education

General education of nursing staff will lead to a better practical understanding of the drugs and techniques used (including simple techniques); the early recognition and treatment of side effects; the physiological and psychological benefits of better acute pain management; and the importance of patient education.

Specialized education

Specialized education leads to safe and effective understanding and management of more sophisticated methods of pain relief such as patient-controlled, epidural, intrathecal or interpleural analgesia.

ACCREDITATION AND REACCREDITATION

Many institutions require some form of certification or accreditation before registered nurses can assume responsibility for a patient whose pain is being managed using one of the specialized methods of pain relief listed above. Accreditation programs usually consist of:

- verbal and written information (e.g. lectures or workshops and booklet)
- written assessment (e.g. multiple choice questionnaire)
- practical assessment (e.g. demonstration of ability to program machines, administer epidural bolus doses)

Reaccreditation every 1–2 years will ensure that knowledge and practices are updated at regular intervals.

These formal education programs need to be supplemented with informal 'one-on-one' teaching in the ward.

PATIENT EDUCATION

Patient education is very important and can make all the difference between effective and ineffective pain relief. The attitudes and expectations of patients can affect how they react to painful stimuli and what they expect from analgesic therapy.

Information should be given to each patient and tailored to the needs of that patient. It should include:

- *procedural information*: details of the medical or surgical procedure
- *sensory information*: descriptions of the sensory experiences that a patient may expect
- *physiological coping information*: instructions for coping with pain related to activities such as coughing and walking

Adequate education and information can lead to decreases in analgesic use and perceptions of pain intensity. For some, however, especially patients with high levels of anxiety or a tendency to use denial or avoidance to deal with problems, excessive information and the need to make decisions can exacerbate anxiety and pain.

Information can be presented in a number of ways, e.g. verbally, in a booklet or on a video. In general, a mix of these methods probably gives the best results. Although education about pain management should ideally start before it is needed, this will not always be possible, for example after an emergency operation or trauma. Regardless of the timing of the initial information, it will often need to be repeated a number of times after analgesic treatment has commenced.

The education requirements for patients are twofold – general and specialized.

GENERAL EDUCATION

Treatment goals and benefits

Patients should know why good analgesia is important for their recovery as well as their comfort. The benefits of physiotherapy and early mobilization should be explained. They should be assured that every attempt will be made to make them as comfortable as possible but that pain scores of zero at all times are usually not achievable with medications currently available. Patients should be told that it is easier to treat pain early than to leave it until it is severe.

Options available for the treatment of acute pain

The options that are available for the treatment of acute pain will vary from case to case but patients should play an active role in expressing their preference after possible risks, benefits and side effects have been explained.

Monitoring pain and its treatment

The reasons for and methods used in the measurement of pain should be outlined. Patients should know that there is no 'right or wrong' answer for pain scores but that these scores are helpful for tailoring analgesic requirements to each patient. In some patients it may be helpful to explain that excessive sedation means that they need a little less opioid.

The need to communicate inadequate analgesia or side effects to staff

Patients should be encouraged to work with their doctors and nurses and to let them know if analgesia is inadequate or if they are experiencing any side effects. If intermittent opioid regimens are being used, the importance of asking for the next dose as soon as they begin to feel uncomfortable should be explained. They should not feel they are 'bothering busy nursing staff'.

Concerns about the risks of addiction

Many patients (or their relatives) are still concerned about the risks of addiction to opioids. Repeated explanations may be required to allay these fears.

SPECIALIZED EDUCATION

Brief explanation of the technique

Explanations of patient-controlled and epidural analgesia should be given including expected duration of therapy and subsequent analgesic management. The description of PCA does not have to be excessively detailed (e.g. explanations of a 5-minute lock-out have led to patients believing that the demand button needs to be pressed every 5 minutes!) The patients must, however, know that they can press the button whenever they are uncomfortable and that they are the only ones allowed to do this (i.e. family and staff are not permitted to do so). Patients should be assured that, despite the use of these techniques, direct personal contact time with nursing staff will not be reduced.

Possible complications and side effects

The safety of PCA and 'being in control' needs to be emphasized. Most of the complications of PCA therapy will be due to the opioids, although an explanation of other causes of some side effects may be useful. For example, patients experiencing nausea or vomiting after bowel surgery may be reluctant to use PCA if they have been told that this is due to the opioid.

The possible side effects and complications of epidural analgesia also should be explained, including the need to report to the hospital immediately if increasing back pain or neurological symptoms occur *after* discharge.

The Agency for Health Care Policy and Research (US Department of Health and Human Services) has issued a booklet titled *Pain Control after Surgery: A Patient's Guide* (Carr et al, 1992). The booklet is in the public domain and the non-copyright information is reproduced in the appendix at the end of this chapter. An example of more specific information given to patients about PCA and epidural analgesia is also included in this appendix.

REFERENCES AND FURTHER READING

Carr D.B., Jacox A.K., Chapman C.R. et al. (1992) Acute Pain Management Guideline Panel. *Pain Control after Surgery. A Patient's Guide.* AHCPR Pub. No. 92-0021. Rockville, MD: Agency for Health Care Policy and Research, Public Health Service, US Department of Health and Human Services.

Carr D.B., Jacox A.K., Chapman C.R. et al. (1992) *Acute Pain Management: Operative or Medical Procedures and Trauma, Clinical Practice Guideline.* AHCPR

Pub. No. 92-0032. Rockville, MD: Agency for Health Care Policy and Research, Public Health Service, US Department of Health and Human Services.

Fields H.L. (ed.) (1991) *Core Curriculum for Professional Education in Pain.* IASP Publications, Seattle.

Owen H., McMillan V. and Rogowski D. (1990) Postoperative pain therapy: a survey of patient's expectations and their experiences. *Pain* **41**, 303–307.

Wilder-Smith C. and Schuler L. (1992) Postoperative analgesia: pain by choice? The influence of patient attitudes and patient education. *Pain* **50**, 257–262.

APPENDIX

Examples of patient information leaflets

9A *Pain Control After Surgery: A Patient Guide,* published by the US Department of Health and Human Services, Rockville, MD, USA.

9B *Patient-Controlled Analgesia (PCA) and Epidural Analgesia* – a patient information sheet published by the Royal Adelaide Hospital Acute Pain Service.

Pain Control After Surgery

A Patient's Guide

The information in this booklet was taken from the *Clinical Practice Guideline for Acute Pain Management: Operative or Medical Procedures and Trauma.* The guideline was developed by a non-Federal expert panel made up of doctors, nurses, other health care providers, an ethicist, and a consumer representative. The guideline a development process was sponsored by the Agency for Health Care Policy and Research (AHCPR), an agency of the U.S. Public Health Service. Other guidelines on common health problems are being developed and a will be released in the near future.

For more information about the guidelines or to receive additional copies of this booklet or other guideline materials, call 1–800–358–9295, or write to the AHCPR Publications Clearinghouse, PO. Box 8547, Silver Spring, MD 20907.

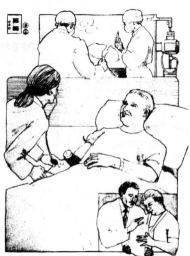

Department of Health and Human Services
Public Health Service
Agency for Health Care Policy and Research
Executive Office Center
2101 East Jefferson Street, Suite 501
Rockville, MD 20852

Pub. No. AHCPR 92-0021

U.S. Department of Health and Human Services
Public Health Service
Agency for Health Care Policy and Research

Pain is an uncomfortable feeling that tells you something may be wrong in your body. Pain is your body's way of sending a warning to your brain. Your spinal cord and nerves provide the pathway for messages to travel to and from your brain and the other parts of your body.

Receptor nerve cells in and beneath your skin sense heat, cold, light, touch, pressure, and pain. You have thousands of these receptor cells, most sense pain and the fewest sense cold. When there is an injury to your body—in this case surgery—these tiny cells send messages along nerves into your spinal cord and then up to your brain. Pain medicine blocks these messages or reduces their effect on your brain.

Sometimes pain may be just a nuisance, like a mild headache. At other times, such as after an operation, pain that doesn't go away—even after you take pain medicine— may be a signal that there is a problem. After your operation, your nurses and doctors will ask you about your pain because they want you to be comfortable, but also because they want to know if something is wrong. Be sure to tell your doctors and nurses when you have pain.

Acute Pain Management Guideline Panel.
Pain Control After Surgery. A Patient's Guide.
AHCPR Pub. No. 92-0021. Rockville, MD:
Agency for Health Care Policy and Research.
Public Health Service, U.S. Department of Health and Human Services. Feb. 1992.

Pain Control After Surgery

A Patient's Guide

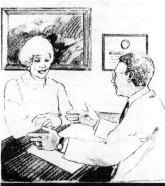

Purpose of this booklet

This booklet talks about pain relief after surgery. It explains the goals of pain control and the types of treatment you may receive. It also shows you how to work with your doctors and nurses to get the best pain control.

Reading the booklet should help you:

- Learn why pain control is important for your recovery as well as your comfort.

- Play an active role in choosing among options for treating your pain.

1

APPENDIX 9A

Treatment Goals

People used to think that severe pain after surgery was something they "just had to put up with." But with current treatments, that's no longer true. Today, you can work with your nurses and doctors before and after surgery to prevent or relieve pain.

Pain control can help you:

- Enjoy greater comfort while you heal.

- Get well faster. With less pain, you can start walking, do your breathing exercises, and get your strength back more quickly. You may even leave the hospital sooner.

- Improve your results. People whose pain is well-controlled seem to do better after surgery. They may avoid some problems (such as pneumonia and blood clots) that affect others.

Pain control: What are the options?

Both drug and non-drug treatments can be successful in helping to prevent and control pain. The most common methods of pain control are described below. You and your doctors and nurses will decide which ones are right for you. Many people combine two or more methods to get greater relief.

Don't worry about getting "hooked" on pain medicines. Studies show that this is very rare—unless you already have a problem with drug abuse.

Pain Control Methods You May Be Using

To get the best results, work with your doctors and nurses to choose the methods that will work best for you.

Your nurses and doctors want to make your surgery as pain free as they can. But you are

the key to getting the best pain relief because pain is personal. The amount or type of pain you feel may not be the same as others feel—even those who have had the same operation.

Before surgery

Drug treatment: Take pain medicine.

Non-drug treatment: Understand what operation the doctor is doing, why it is being done, and how it will be done. Learn how to do deep breathing and relaxation exercises (see example on pages 6 and 7).

During surgery:

Drug treatment: Receive general anesthesia, spinal anesthesia, or nerve blocks, or take a pain medicine through a small tube in your back (called an epidural).

After surgery

Drug treatment: Take a pain medicine as a pill, shot, or suppository, or through a tube in your vein or back.

Non-drug treatment: Use massage, hot or cold packs, relaxation, music or other pastimes to distract you, positive thinking, or nerve stimulation (TENS).

What can you do to help keep your pain under control? These seven steps can help you help yourself.

Before surgery

1 Ask the doctor or nurse what to expect.

- Will there be much pain after surgery?

- Where will it occur?

- How long is it likely to last?

Being prepared helps put you in control. You may want to write down your questions before you meet with your doctor or nurse.

2 Discuss the pain control options on pages 2 and 3 of this booklet with your doctors and nurses.

Be sure to:

- Talk with your nurses and doctors about pain control methods that have worked well or not so well for you before.

- Talk with your nurses and doctors about any concerns you may have about pain medicine.

- Tell your doctors and nurses about any allergies to medicines you may have.

- Ask about side effects that may occur with treatment.

- Talk with your nurses and doctors about the medicines you take for other health problems. The doctors and nurses need to know, because mixing some drugs with some pain medicines can cause problems.

3 Talk about the schedule for pain medicines in the hospital.

Some people get pain medicines in the hospital only when they call the nurse to ask for them. Sometimes there are delays, and the pain gets worse while they wait.

Today, two other ways to schedule pain medicines seem to give better results.

- Giving the pain pills or shots at set times. Instead of waiting until pain breaks through, you receive medicine at set times during the day to keep the pain under control.

- Patient controlled analgesia (PCA) may be available in your hospital. With PCA, you control when you get pain medicine. When you begin to feel pain, you press a button to inject the medicine through the intravenous (IV) tube in your vein.

For both ways, your nurses and doctors will ask you how the pain medicine is working and change the medicine, its dose, or its timing if you are still having pain.

4 Work with your doctors and nurses to make a pain control plan.

You can use the form on pages 12 and 13 to begin planning for pain control with your nurses and doctors. They need your help to design the best plan for you. When your pain control plan is complete, use the form to write down what will happen. Refer to it after your operation. Then keep it as a record if you need surgery in the future.

After surgery

5 Take (or ask for) pain relief drugs when pain first begins.

- Take action as soon as the pain starts.

- If you know your pain will worsen when you start working or doing breathing exercises, take pain medicine first. It's harder to ease pain once it has taken hold.

This is a key step in proper pain control.

6 Help the doctors and nurses "measure" your pain.

- They may ask you to rate your pain on a scale of 0 to 10. Or you may choose a word from a list that best describes the pain.

- You may also set a pain control goal (such as having no pain that's worse than 2 on the scale).

- Reporting your pain as a number helps the doctors and nurses know how well your treatment is working and whether to make any changes.

- They may ask you to use a "pain scale" like the one shown on page 7.

4

5

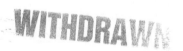

APPENDIX 9A

7 Tell the doctor or nurse about any pain that won't go away.

- Don't worry about being a "bother."
- Pain can be a sign of problems with your operation.
- The nurses and doctors want and need to know about it.

Stick with your pain control plan if it's working. Your doctors and nurses can change the plan if your pain is not under control. You need to tell the nurses and doctors about your pain and how the pain control plan is working.

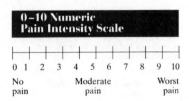

0–10 Numeric Pain Intensity Scale

0	1	2	3	4	5	6	7	8	9	10

No pain   Moderate pain   Worst pain

APPENDIX 9A

Benefits and Risks of Pain Treatment Methods

This information is provided to help you discuss your options with your doctors and nurses. Sometimes it is best to combine two or more of these treatments or change the treatments slightly to meet your individual needs. Your doctors and nurses will discuss this with you.

Pain Relief Medicines

Nonsteroidal anti-inflammatory drugs: Acetaminophen (for example, Tylenol), aspirin, ibuprofen (for example, Motrin), and other NSAIDs reduce swelling and soreness and relieve mild to moderate pain.

Benefits: There is no risk of addiction to these medicines. Depending on how much pain you have, these medicines can lessen or eliminate the need for stronger medicines (for example, morphine or another opioid).

Risks: Most NSAIDs interfere with blood clotting. They may cause nausea, stomach bleeding, or kidney problems. For severe pain, an opioid usually must be added.

Opioids: Morphine, codeine, and other opioids are most often used for acute pain, such as short-term pain after surgery.

Benefits: These medicines are effective for severe pain, and they do not cause bleeding in the stomach or elsewhere. It is rare for a patient to become addicted as a result of taking opioids for postoperative pain.

Risks: Opioids may cause drowsiness, nausea, constipation, itching, or interfere with breathing or urination.

Local anesthetics: These drugs (for example, bupivacaine) are given, either near the incision or through a small tube in your back, to block the nerves that transmit pain signals.

Benefits: Local anesthetics are effective for severe pain. Injections at the incision site block pain from that site. There is little or no risk of drowsiness, constipation, or breathing problems. Local anesthetics reduce the need for opioid use.

Risks: Repeated injections are needed to maintain pain relief. An overdose of local anesthetic can have serious consequences. Average doses may cause some patients to have weakness in their legs or dizziness.

Methods Used to Give Pain Relief Medicines

Tablet or liquid: Medicines given by mouth (for example, aspirin, ibuprofen, or opioid medications such as codeine).

Benefits: Tablets and liquids cause less discomfort than injections into muscle or skin, but they can work just as well. They are inexpensive, simple to give, and easy to use at home.

Risks: These medicines cannot be used if nothing can be taken by mouth or if you are nauseated or vomiting; sometimes these medicines can be given rectally (suppository form). There may be a delay in pain relief, since you must ask for the medicine and wait for it to be brought to you; also, these medicines take time to wear off.

8

9

APPENDIX 9A

Injections into skin or muscle

Benefits: Medicine given by injection into skin or muscle is effective even if you are nauseated or vomiting; such injections are simple to give.

Risks: The injection site is usually painful for a short time. Medicines given by injection are more expensive than tablets or liquids and take time to wear off. Pain relief may be delayed while you ask the nurse for medicine and wait for the shot to be drawn up and given.

Injections into vein:
Pain relief medicines are injected into a vein through a small tube, called an intravenous (IV) catheter. The tip of the tube stays in the vein.

Benefits: Medicines given by injection into a vein are fully absorbed and act quickly. This method is well suited for relief of brief episodes of pain. When a patient controlled analgesia (PCA) pump is used, you can control your own doses of pain medicine.

Risks: A small tube must be inserted in a vein. If PCA is used, there are extra costs for pumps, supplies, and staff training. You must want to use the pump and learn how and when to give yourself doses of medicine.

Injections into spine:
Medicine is given through a small tube in your back (called an epidural or intrathecal catheter).

Benefits: This method works well when you have chest surgery or an operation on the lower parts of your body.

Risks: Staff must be specially trained to place a small tube in the back and to watch for problems that can appear hours after pain medicine is given. Extra cost is involved for staff time and training and to purchase pumps and supplies.

Non-drug Pain Relief Methods

These methods can be effective for mild to moderate pain and to boost the pain-relief effects of drugs. There are no side effects. These techniques are best learned before surgery.

Patient teaching: Learning about the operation and the pain expected afterwards (for example, when coughing or getting out of bed or a chair).

Benefits: These techniques can reduce anxiety; they are simple to learn, and no equipment is needed.

Risks: There are no risks; however, patient attention and cooperation with staff are required.

Relaxation: Simple techniques, such as abdominal breathing and jaw relaxation, can help to increase your comfort after surgery.

Benefits: Relaxation techniques are easy to learn, and they can help to reduce anxiety. After instruction, you can use relaxation at any time. No equipment is needed.

Risks: There are no risks, but you will need instruction from your nurse or doctor.

Physical agents: Cold packs, massage, rest, and TENS therapy are some of the non-drug pain relief methods that might be used following surgery.

Benefits: In general, physical agents are safe and have no side effects. TENS, which stands for transcutaneous electrical nerve stimulation, is often helpful; it is quick to act and can be controlled by the patient.

Risks: There are no risks related to the use of physical techniques for managing pain. If TENS is used, there is some cost and staff time involved for purchasing the machine and instructing patients in its use. Also, there is only limited evidence to support the effectiveness of TENS for pain relief in certain situations.

10

11

1/1/93

> Acute Pain Service
> Royal Adelaide Hospital
>
> ## PATIENT INFORMATION
>
> ### PATIENT-CONTROLLED ANALGESIA (PCA)
> ### AND EPIDURAL ANALGESIA

The management of acute pain, particularly pain following more major operations or accidents, has improved quite significantly over the past few years. No longer are injections into your arm or leg the only way of giving strong pain killing drugs.

You may be offered one of these new pain relieving methods to help treat your pain. Here at the Royal Adelaide Hospital the two most commonly used of these methods are **patient-controlled analgesia** (called PCA for short) and **epidural analgesia.**

Analgesia means "painlessness" or "no pain". Unfortunately, with the drugs that are currently available, it is usually *not* possible to safely relieve *all* the pain. Instead, we aim for enough pain relief to make you *comfortable*, so that you can sleep, move around and, very importantly, do coughing and deep breathing and other physiotherapy exercises.

The **Acute Pain Service (APS)** is part of the Department of Anaesthesia at the Royal Adelaide Hospital. Anaesthetists are the doctors who look after your anaesthetic during your operation, but they also specialise in pain relief. If you have one of the newer forms of pain relief you will be seen at least once a day by an anaesthetist and nurse from the APS in addition the doctors and nurses who provide your regular ward care. The APS also has an anaesthetist on-call 24 hours a day.

Is pain relief important?
Yes. As well as making patients more comfortable, good pain relief can help speed recovery. This is especially true for patients having more major operations.

APPENDIX 9B

PATIENT-CONTROLLED ANALGESIA (PCA)

PCA means that you actually have control over your own pain relief. There is a machine called a PCA pump that can be used to give a small dose of a strong pain killer, such as morphine or pethidine. Usually this machine will be attached to the drip (intravenous line) in your arm. If you are uncomfortable you press a button and the machine will pump a small dose of the drug into this line. You can do this whenever you are uncomfortable - you do not need to tell the nurse first. The amount of drug delivered by the machine each time you press the button, as well as other settings on the machine, will be ordered by the anaesthetist from the Acute Pain Service. The PCA machine will be programmed by your nurse according to these orders.

How often can I press the button?
You can press the PCA button whenever you feel uncomfortable. However, once the button has been pushed and the PCA machine has delivered the dose (this takes about 1 minute) the machine will "lockout" for 5 minutes. This means that, even if you push the button within this "lockout" time of 5 minutes, the PCA machine will not respond. This is so that you have time to feel the effect of one dose of pain relieving drug before getting another dose. Remember, the aim is to make yourself comfortable - it is not always possible to be completely pain free.

Who is allowed to press the PCA button?
The patient is the ONLY person allowed to press the button. Do not allow ANY hospital staff, relatives or friends to do so.

Will the pain relieving drug work immediately?
No. These drugs need to get to the brain and spinal cord and it may take 5 minutes or longer for the drug to work fully. However, this is still much quicker than if these drugs were given by injection into your arm or leg. If you are about to do something that you know will hurt, like coughing or moving, press the PCA button about 5 minutes *before* doing it.

What if the pain relieving drug doesn't work?
If you are pressing the PCA button quite frequently and are still uncomfortable tell your nurse, who will firstly check that the drip is running properly. As long as you are not sleepy your nurse can increase the

APPENDIX 9B

1/1/93

amount of drug you get when you press the button. If necessary, the Acute Pain Service will be consulted.

Can I overdose?
PCA is probably one of the safest ways of giving strong pain killing drugs. The dose of drug that you get with each press of the button is very small so if you were getting just a little too much you would feel sleepy. This means that you would not press the button again. Your nurse would also notice this and would reduce the amount of drug delivered with each push of the button and, if necessary, treat the sleepiness. The amount of pain relieving drug that is needed varies greatly between patients so it is not unusual to have to make alterations in the dose.

Can I get addicted?
When drugs like morphine and pethidine are used to treat acute pain like the pain after operations or accidents, the risk of addiction is negligible. It is very important *not* to let the fear of addiction stop you from using enough of the drugs to be comfortable or to stop you from moving or coughing.

Will I feel nauseated or vomit?
There are many reasons for feeling sick after operations - drugs like morphine and pethidine are only one possible cause. Whatever the cause, you will be ordered other drugs called *antiemetics* that can help counteract the nausea or vomiting. If one of these drugs doesn't work your nurse will try another. If the morphine or pethidine does seem to be causing the problem, or at least making it worse, it is often because the dose of the drug is a little high. There doesn't seem to be a great difference between these two drugs and for this reason we will often decrease the dose that you get from each press of the PCA button, or increase the time the PCA machine takes to deliver the drug. Occasionally, it may help to change the drug.

For how long will I use PCA?
Normally PCA will continue while you have your drip in. When your doctors on the ward allow you to drink it means that the drip may soon be removed. PCA will usually stop at this time but you will be ordered other pain relieving drugs should you need them. Commonly these pain killers will be tablets. The type and number of tablets will depend of how much pain relieving drug you used with PCA.

APPENDIX 9B

EPIDURAL ANALGESIA

You may already know about epidural analgesia as it is a method often used to treat pain during childbirth. This same technique can also be used to treat pain after some operations and accidents. Most pain relieving drugs work by acting on the brain and spinal cord and they are carried there in the blood stream. With an epidural, the use of a very small plastic tube means that these drugs can be placed close to the spinal cord and nerves so that the drugs can act directly on them and not have to travel to them in the blood stream. This method of pain relief is one of the best available but it is not necessary after all operations or accidents. If you have an epidural for pain relief it will be put in by your anaesthetist, who will explain the procedure to you beforehand.

What pain relieving drugs are used with an epidural?
Two types of drugs are used - drugs like morphine and pethidine or drugs called local anaesthetics. Most often we use a mixture of the two types of drugs.

What if the epidural doesn't work?
If you are uncomfortable tell your nurse who will check the epidural and can increase the amount of drug that you are getting. If necessary, the Acute Pain Service may also be contacted.

Will my legs feel numb, weak or heavy?
If you are having an operation, the epidural will often be used as part of the anaesthetic as well as for pain relief afterwards. A strong local anaesthetic drug may be given during the operation so immediately after the operation your legs may feel numb and heavy. This will wear off in a few hours. The drugs that we use for pain relief in an epidural after the operation will not be as strong so your legs should feel virtually normal. If they do not, let your nurse know. The aim is to keep you comfortable but still able to move around in bed, sit out of bed and even walk, if your doctors allow it.

Will my legs be numb, weak or heavy when I leave hospital?
NO. In the unlikely event that you have gone home and notice persistent tingling, numbness, heaviness or weakness in your legs, or have trouble passing water, or have a pain in your back that is getting worse, you should tell your doctor immediately and ask him/her to contact the APS at the Royal Adelaide Hospital.

Numbers in *italic* refer to illustrations or tables.
Numbers in **bold** refer to main discussion.

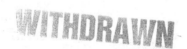